Guidelines and Screening Methods of Pharmacology

An Essential Guide To Pharmacy and Life Sciences Research Scholars

Guidelines and Screening Methods of Pharmacology

An Essential Guide To Pharmacy and Life Sciences Research Scholars

Surendra H. Bodakhe

M.Pharm., Ph.D, FIC

Associate Professor of Pharmacology,
SLT Institute of Pharmaceutical Sciences, Guru Ghasidas Vishwavidyalaya
(A Central University), Bilaspur (Chattisgarh).

Parag Jain

Assistant Professor,
CSIT, Bhilai, Chattisgarh.

Arin Bhattacharya

Assistant Professor,
JK college of Pharmacy, Bilaspur (Chattisgarh).

Jaya Shree

M.Pharm., Ph.D.

Assistant Professor,
Rungta Institute of Pharmaceutical Sciences (SRGI), Bhilai, (Chattisgarh).

Amrita Singh

Ph.D research scholar,
SLT Institute of Pharmaceutical Sciences, Guru Ghasidas Vishwavidyalaya
(A Central University), Bilaspur (Chattisgarh).

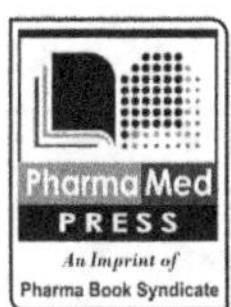

PharmaMed Press

An imprint of Pharma Book Syndicate
A unit of BSP Books Pvt. Ltd.
4-4-309/316, Giriraj Lane,
Sultan Bazar, Hyderabad - 500 095.

Guidelines and Screening Methods of Pharmacology

by Surendra H. Bodakhe, Parag Jain, Arin Bhattacharya, Jaya Shree and Amrita Singh

Published by

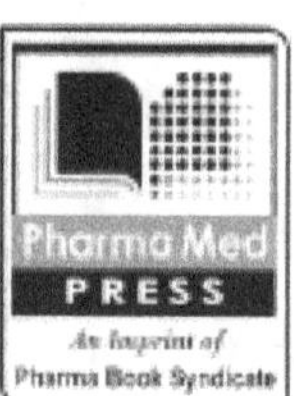

PharmaMed Press

An imprint of Pharma Book Syndicate

A unit of BSP Books Pvt. Ltd.

4-4-309/316, Giriraj Lane, Sultan Bazar, Hyderabad - 500 095.
Phone: 040-23445688; Fax: 91+40-23445611
e-mail: info@pharmamedpress.com
www.pharmamedpress.com/pharmamedpress.net

ISBN: 978-93-89354-60-7

PREFACE

Pharmacological screening of drugs is the sequential testing of new chemical entities or extracts from biological material in isolated organs followed by test in whole animals. Therefore, it is of utmost importance to describe the pharmacological screening methods in order to maximize the benefits and optimize the risks of drugs to recipients. The student in pharmacology, the pharmacist and the medicinal chemist will find a survey of pharmacological assays that can be used for a given indication and for which methods have demonstrated their relevance. However, this book will also be useful for other health professionals whose career involves testing of biological activity of drugs. The goal is to empower the students through an understanding the basic models for screening the biological activity of drug. Certain therapeutic domains, such as cardiovascular, respiratory and renal disorders, psychiatry and neurology, peripheral nerve function, pain and rheumatic diseases, metabolic and endocrine diseases including diseases of the gastrointestinal tract, are discussed in this book. Each chapter is divided into pharmacological classes, e.g., anxiolytics, antiepileptics, neuroleptics, antidepressants, or anti-Parkinson drugs in central nervous system; bronchodilators, expectorants, antiasthmatic and antispasmodics in respiratory system. For each class, *in vitro* methods, tests on isolated organs and *in vivo* methods are described. For each method the purpose and rationale are given first, followed by a description of the procedure, evaluation of the data, modifications of the method described in the literature, and the relevant references. Wherever possible, a critical assessment of the method based on personal experience is added. The guidelines concerning the care and use of laboratory animals have been updated. Readers are encouraged to refer the references mentioned for further information and we hope that this book will be a valuable companion in our pursuit of a fundamental understanding of experimental models in a most fascinating area of screening pharmacology.

- Authors

CONTENTS

CHAPTER 1

Regulations for Laboratory Animals Care and Ethical Requirements

CHAPTER 2

Pharmacological Techniques for Evaluation of Drugs on Different Systems

CHAPTER 3

Bioassay

CHAPTER 4

Evaluation of Drugs acting on Autonomic Nervous System

CHAPTER 5

Evaluation of Drugs Acting on Central Nervous System

CHAPTER 6

Evaluation of Drugs Acting on Respiratory System

CHAPTER 7

Evaluation of Drugs Acting on Eye

CHAPTER 8

Evaluation of Drugs Acting on Cardiovascular System

Chapter 9

Evaluation of Drugs Acting on Endocrine System

Chapter 10

Evaluation of Drug Acting on Kidney

CHAPTER 11

Miscellaneous

CHAPTER 12

Transgenic Animals and other Genetically Modified Animal Models

CHAPTER 13

Drug Toxicity and Safety Evaluation

CHAPTER 14

Alternatives to Animal Screening Procedures

CHAPTER 15

New Approaches in Drug Discovery

CHAPTER 16

Research Methodology

Chapter 1

Regulations for Laboratory Animals Care and Ethical Requirements

1.1 Introduction

Animal ethics includes all the specifications required to treat animal in a generous way and it ensures that minimum pain should be given to them. In 1959, William Russell and Rex Burch gave; the 3R's principles (based on reduction, refinement and replacement of animals) of Humane Experimental Technique, the scientific excellence and humane use of laboratory animals.

- **Reduction:** Use less number of animals, different group of animals can be combined together with colleagues and thus results can be obtained from less number of animals.

- **Refinement:** Use techniques to decrease pain/suffering, alteration in frequency and volume of dose, improvement of animal well-being.

- **Replacement:** Use techniques that substitute organisms with isolated organs, microorganisms, invertebrates, and sometimes mathematics and computer models.

- Previously, it was 3R's principles but now one more principle is added and it is known as 4R's principles "reuse".

- **Reuse:** Resuse of same animals in other experiments after approval from competent authority like Institutional Animal Ethics Committee (IAEC).

1.2 Committee for the Purpose of Control and Supervision of Experiments on Animals (CPCSEA)

A committee is shaped with the main aim to explore all such requirement that may be essential to guarantee that animals are not given any kind of pain before, during or after the experiment known as Committee for the

Purpose of Control and Supervision of Experiments on Animals (CPCSEA). This legal body is work according to Prevention of Cruelty to Animals Act, 1960 which is currently under the Ministry of Fisheries, Animal husbandry and dairying department of India. Various norms have been prepared by this committee to maintain quality and safety of animals. It plays role in regulation of experimental studies for proper conduction of biomedical and behavioral research along with testing of products.

1.2.1 Goal

The main aim of CPCSEA guidelines is to promote proper care of animals that is used during experiments. The major objective is to provide specifications that will improve animal well-being. It is also helpful in the search of advancement of biological knowledge that is pertinent to animals and humans.

1.2.2 Principles Adopted by CPCSEA for Animal Experimentation

- Experiments be performed on animals with the intention of progress of new drugs or discovery of physiologic knowledge that is predictable to be useful for protecting or prolonging human life or preventing suffering or against any disease, whether of human being, animals or plants.

- The selection of animals for the experiment should be based on lowest phylogenetic scale that may produce scientifically valid results. Experimental protocol must be intended in such a manner to allow minimum number of animals to provide statistically valid results at 95% level of confidence.

  [**Note:** Phylogenetic scale- animals are ranked according to their general complexity and ability from lowest to highest. Research protocols should be prepared in such a way that experiments on animals rank lower on the phylogenetic scale. Rodents are lower on the scale than any other animal species].

- It should be the main concern to use experimental animals properly and to prevent and reduce pain and suffering inflicted on animals.

- Welfare of animals after their use in experiments must be the moral responsibility of research personnel engaged in animal experimentation. It is the responsibility of researchers for care and rehabilitation of animals after experiments. The animals are permitted to euthanize after study.

[**Note:** Euthanasia should be given to animals in following conditions when animal is paralyzed and unable to perform daily functions, locomotion, pain and suffering from long time and other life threatening conditions to human beings or other animals].

- Proper housing, feeding and caring of animals should be maintained. The conditions of living for animals should be comfortable.

[**Note:** For proper caring, handling and use of the animal species in biomedical research a veterinarian or a scientist engaged in animal experimentation must be appointed].

1.2.3 Functions of CPCSEA

The following are the functions of CPCSEA:

- The organization or institute engaged in animal experimentation or breeding of animals should be registered.

- Appointment of nominees for IAEC.

- Approve any establishment or institute having animal house facilities on the basis of reports of inspections.

  Note: CPCSEA team may conduct both announced and unannounced visits to the registered establishments for the inspection of the animal house facilities in the institutes.

- To give permission for proper conduction of animals experiments on animals.

- Recommendations for import of animals for use in experiments.

- Committee can take any legal action against establishment or suspend their registration in case of violation of principles and guidelines.

- Any institution or establishment registered under CPCSEA must constitute Institutional Animals Ethics Committee (IAEC). IAEC is an organization comprised of a group of recognized persons and registered by the committee for the purpose and supervision of experiments on animals in an establishment. IAEC includes eight members Figure 1.1 depicts about composition of IAEC.

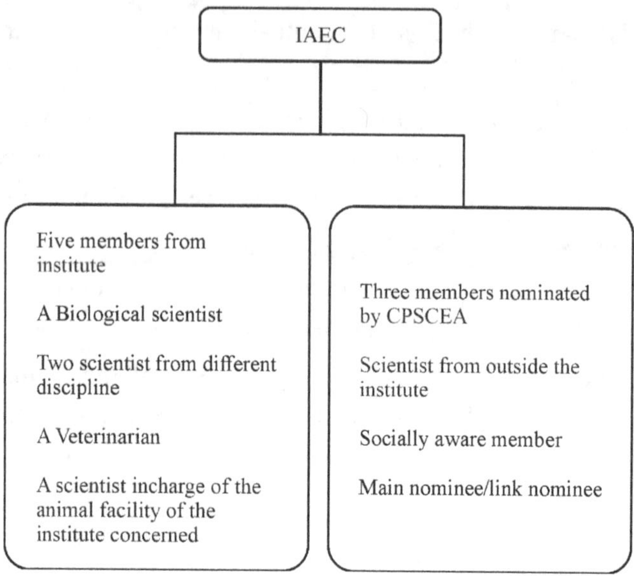

Figure 1.1 Constitution of IAEC.

1. *Five members from establishment or institute:* (two scientists from different biological disciplines, one biological scientist, one veterinarian involved in the case of animal, one scientist in charge of the animal facility of the institute concerned).

2. *Three members nominated by CPSCEA:* socially aware member (1), scientist from other institute (1), main nominee (1) and Link nominee (*)

   Link Nominee shall substitute the main nominee in case main nominee conveys his unavailability in writing to the chairperson of the IAEC in advance as per described procedure.

1.2.4 Functions of IAEC

- IAEC will come across and grant permission against feasible and appropriate proposal involving animals experimentation before start of the study. In case of proposal containing large number of animals the IAEC must forward it to CPCSEA in prescribed format with prescribed manner with its recommendation.

- IAEC gives permission for experiments on small animals only up to the phylogenetic scale of rodents. The committee does not have authority to approve any research proposal involving animals higher on the phylogenetic scale than rodents.

Note: The committee may consider such type of proposal involving animals above sentience level of rodents, and then forward the proposal to CPCSEA for its recommendations.

- Research activities performed in any institution must be governed by IAEC periodically and after completion of study. IAEC visits the organization performing animal experiments from time to time.

- The IAEC committee is also abide to other compliances, regulatory requirements, rules and guidelines specified by CPCSEA.

  Note: IAEC is appointed for the period of 5 years (earlier it was for 3 years) and it can be reconstituted at the time of renewal of registration, if required.

1.2.5 CPCSEA Guidelines for Laboratory Animals

CPCSEA has prepared certain guidelines for welfare of animals to promote proper care of animals used in biomedical and behavioral research. Every establishment must obey these guidelines including Good Laboratory Practices (GLP) engaged in animal experimentation to assure quality maintenance and well-being of laboratory animals while conducting experiments research and testing of products. Different parameters need to fulfill or take in consideration according to these guidelines are:

(a) Veterinary care

It is the responsibility of a veterinarian or a person appointed in the institute having experience in laboratory animal handling for adequate care of animals. Animals should be observed daily by someone other than a veterinarian and communicate timely with veterinarian regarding well-being of animals or any problems in animal health and behavior. The veterinarian can participate in reviewing protocols and proposals, monitoring of occupational health hazards and control of zoonosis. Individual can establish appropriate guidelines for veterinary care, animal husbandry and animal welfare, supervising animal nutrition and sanitation.

(b) Animal procurement

All animals should be procured ethically from the registered breeder as per the guidelines of CPCSEA. The procured animals should be assessed carefully regarding its healthiness and it should be devoid of any diseases. A health surveillance program may be there to screen incoming animals. Animals should be quarantined, stabilized and separated according to procedure appropriate for the particular circumstances and species.

(c) Quarantine

Quarantine means how the new animals are kept in their housing. They must be separated from old animals .The health of the animals must be checked for any kind of infection. Time for quarantine may be a week; month or more than a month depends upon phylogenetic arrangement of the animals.

(d) Stabilization

New animals must stabilize physiologically, psychologically and nutritionally. Period of stabilization depends upon the animal's transportation duration, type of species and type of animals use.

(e) Separation

Separation should be done according to species. Separation is mainly done to inhibit disease transfer from one species to another species. It eliminates anxiety, behavioral and physiological changes due to interspecies conflict. For different groups of animals different personnel must be appointed. No other personnel should be allowed to enter the area.

(f) Monitoring, Diagnosis and Control of Disease

Animals should be kept in examination by a competent staff. Animals should be watched daily but if the animal is sick or any experiment is carried out to that particular animal then that animal must be observed carefully. Animal must be given veterinary care if needed at the proper time. If the animal is suffering from infection then it must be kept isolated from others. If bacterial infection persists in the entire room then the animal group should be kept separate and isolated during the process of observation, treatment and control.

(g) Animal care and Technical personnel

The staff trained in laboratory animal science can only be appointed by the institution for animal care. Institution may provide formal or on-job training to assure about the trained staff. Staff engaged in animal care must be aware of hygiene and must maintain cleanliness. Personnel protective equipment (PPE) like footwear, gloves, masks, coats, head covers; cloths etc. must be provided to reach the animal house to maintain cleanliness. PPE must be free of dust, toxic elements. Eating, drinking, smoking should be banned inside the animal house.

(h) Animal experimentation involving hazardous agent

Institutions engaged in testing of hazardous agents on animals must constitute a Bio-safety committee for taking care of safety issues. Bio safety committee must check the proposals in those protocols which are using hazardous substance.

(i) Duration of experiment

In most of the cases animal should be used for experiment only for 3 years but in special cases it can be used for more than 3 years.

(j) Physical restrain

Equipment used to perform experimental design should be carefully designed so that least pain is given to animals. The period of restraint should be less. Animals are given prior training before experiment to minimize stress. Veterinarian should be there to avoid any kind of infection during experiment.

(k) Physical facilities

Animal facilities should be well planned, properly maintained and comfortable to the animals. It may vary according to the design and size to the institute, in-house animal and geographical location. The building materials used for construction of building should be moisture-resistant, durable, fire-resistant, seamless material and vermin/ pest control. Sufficient corridor space should be provided for movement of personnel and handling of equipment. Other facilities including water lines, drain pipes and electrical connections should be provided.

(l) Location of animal house

Animals must be housed in a place which is far away from the human activities for proper animal husbandry, human comfort and protection of health. Following steps should be taken into consideration:

- Animal house should be situated at a distance from human residence and it should be free from ticks, smoke, dust, noise, insects, wild rodents and birds.

- Nearby laboratories should be adequately separated using barriers such as entry locks, corridors or floors.

- Animal shelter should occupy approx. 50-60% of total constructed area; however, the remaining area should be utilized for other services like washing, stores, staff, office and quarantine, machine rooms and corridors.

- Animals should remain free from fluctuating environment, temperature, light, humidity, sound and ventilation, as animals are very sensitive to these factors.

(m) Infrastructures

Animal house doors should fit appropriately, so that the room should be free from rust, vermin and dust. Windows are optional for small animal facilities. There must be arrangement of alternate source of light and ventilation in-case of power failures and backup power is not available. Floors should remain dry. It should not absorb anything. It should be free from skid, resistant to acid, wear, solvents, adverse effects of disinfectants and detergents. It should be sufficiently strong to bear weight of racks, equipment and stored items. Walls and ceiling should be free of cracks, seepage, or damaged junctions with floors, doors and corners. Construction material should be capable to withstand on scrubbing with disinfectants, detergents and under high pressure of water.

(n) Environmental conditions

Temperature of the animal house is kept at 18-29°C and humidity of the animal house is 30% to 70% RH. Air conditioning is valuable means of regulating these environmental conditions. Ventilation system should be designed in such a way to allow 12-15 air cycles per hour. Power and lighting system should be maintained as 12 h light and 12 h dark cycle. Animal house must be made of concrete walls to avoid noise pollution. Allowed sound for rodents and non-human primates is 85 dB.

(o) Animal husbandry

Animal husbandry should be planned carefully for facilitation of animal well-being, to meet research requirements to minimize experimental variable. Cages allow meeting the biological needs of the animals like maintenance of body temperature, urination, defecation and reproduction. Cages are generally made of polypropylene, polycarbonate and stainless steel. Cage surface should be smooth and impermeable so it should not pull or keep dirt.

(p) Caging or Housing System

Caging of animals plays a vital role in social and physical behavior of animals. It should be designed appropriately for more comfort to the animals. The housing of cage animals should possess following facilities:

- Adequate space, liberty to move and adjustments of normal posture, and a resting place for appropriateness of the species.

- Provide a comfortable environment to the animals.

- Provide no escape for the animals from the cages which confines animal safety.

- Provision of food and water to the animals, must be easy.

- Provide proper ventilation.

- Confirm the biological requirement of the animals, e.g., maintenance of body temperature, urination, defecation, and reproduction.

- In cages, animals must be maintained dry and clean.

- Increase research possibility while maintaining good health of the animals.

  The caging of the animals should be made up of tough materials, strong, and designed in such a manner that cross-infection between adjoining units should be very minimum. Cages of polycarbonate, polypropylene and stainless steel should be used for laboratory animals. Cages of animals like monkeys, sheep and horses should be made up of steel or painted mild steel. Cages should be clean and impermeable with smooth surface. The animals can be seen clearly from outside the cages without disturbing to them.

Feeding and watering devices should be clean. Handling should be easy for these devices. Cages should be comfortable to prevent injuries to animals with regular cleaning and servicing.

(q) Sheltered or Outdoor Housing

Few animals are kept outside. They are kept in runs, pens, or large enclosure. There must be proper defense mechanism to prevent from high temperature or harsh weather conditions and adequate protective escape mechanism for animals such as monkeys. Protection should be given to all animals. Proper ventilation must be there. The furnitures must be replaceable in conditions of soiled and worn out. The ground level of the housing facilities should be covered with sand, gravel, grass, absorbent bedding and other material that can be replaced or removed when needed to insure sanitation.

(r) Social Environment

The social environment is the surrounding of the animals among group of individuals to communicate. It may vary according to species and experiences of the animals. While keeping the animal in a particular environment or social interaction, the natural habitat and behavior of the animals should be kept in mind either to place single or in a group. During grouping of animals their sex, age, and social rank should be studied. Population density can affect the metabolism, behavior, reproduction and immune responses. The group composition should be constant for non-human primates, canine and other large mammals to avoid behavioral and physiological changes.

1.3   Euthanasia

Euthanasia is also popularly known as "mercy killing". Euthanasia is the least painful death given to animal after the end of the experiment. If the animals are experiencing severe pain during the experiment then those animals are euthanized to relieve the pain. There are various types of euthanasia methods. These methods are species specific and must be appropriate for particular research. American Veterinary Medical Association (AVMA) Panel had given various justifications on techniques of Euthanasia. The justification must be given for any deviation from AVMA recommendations. Euthanasia should be performed rapidly and it is performed in a different room in which animals are housed. CPCSEA has also given guidelines for euthanasia.

1.3.1 Inhalant Euthanasia

Inhalant anesthetics are slow in action because after reaching to the alveoli when it attains a certain concentration then it starts its action. Various inhalant anesthetics are ether, sevoflurane, halothane, isoflurane. Inhalation anesthetics produce respiratory and cardiac arrest.

- Halothane is best alternative of sevoflurane in term of cost. However, action of sevoflurane is quick. These agents are safe but it should be used cautiously to avoid exposure to vapors.

- Ether irritates the respiratory tract, causing stress and is explosive hazard therefore not recommended. It should be used under fume hood.

1.3.2 Carbon Dioxide (CO_2)

Carbon dioxide (CO_2) is a good euthanasia used for all animals including rodents. Its concentration should be between 60-70% and exposure time should not be more than 5 min. CO_2 is a reversible anesthetic, its long term exposure causes respiratory arrest.

1.3.3 Non Inhalant Pharmacological Agents

(a) **Barbiturates:** Pentobarbital is barbiturate drug used for birds and mammalian species. It is administered intravenously in animals except rodents; in rodents intraperitoneal route is used for drug administration.

Advantages

- Quick onset of action.
- Barbiturates produce good euthanasia with least distress.
- Barbiturates are cost effective.

Disadvantage

- Barbiturates are used intravenously so it requires skilled personnel.

(b) **Chloral hydrate:** Chloral hydrate suppresses the cerebrum activity. It causes hypoxemia and then death. It is used for large animals.

(c) **Magnesium sulfate or potassium chloride:** Both magnesium sulfate or potassium chloride is used in combination for euthanasia. However, the dose can be enhanced along with potassium chloride in anesthetized animals. Potassium chloride is given in concentrated form to cause cardiac arrest.

(d) **MS 222:** Tricaine methane sulfonate (MS222) is used an euthanasia agent for fish and amphibians. It can be administered through injection (200-300 mg/kg of a 1% buffered solution) or as an immersion bath (2 mg/ml in H_2O, exposed for 20 min to 3 h). However, immersion in benzocaine (100-200 mg/L H_2O) is also acceptable.

[**Note:** Precaution should be taken while handling MS222 to wean gloves all times. It may cause retinal toxicity due to exposure].

1.3.4 Physical Methods

The use of these techniques require experience and skilled personnel.

(a) **Exsanguinations** is performed by giving anesthesia to all animals. It is acceptable to all species.

(b) **Cervical dislocation** is permissible of most of the animals including rats, birds, mice and rabbits, however, it require skill and proper technique to perform. Thus, animals should be anesthetized to do it easily.

(c) **Decapitation technique** is used for birds or small mammals. Carbon dioxide or phenobarbital is used to anesthetize animals. The scientific justification is required for using decapitation technique as a sole means of euthanasia. It is only performed when study required to use this technique because it is hazardous to personnel. The animals are decapitated alone to avoid anxiety to other animals with smell of blood and gloves should be changed between animals. It causes rapid loss of consciousness.

(d) **Pithing** is used as a sole technique of euthanasia for frogs and other amphibians. Pithing is generally followed by decapitation.

(e) **Stunning, rapid freezing or air embolism** is permissible for small species but scientific justification is required and used when no alternatives are available.

1.4   International Conference on Harmonization (ICH)

International Conference on Harmonization (ICH) was created in April 1990 at Brussels. It involves regulators and industry for discussing scientific and technical matters to ensure and assess quality, safety and efficacy of drugs. It was an agreement between the United States of America, Europe and Japan to harmonize different regional requirements for registration of pharmaceutical drug products.

1.4.1 Mission

The guidelines were passed with the aim to achieve greater harmony in the interpretation and application of technical guidelines. It is also subjected to reduce duplicity of testing during research and development of new drugs.

1.4.2 Objectives

The main objective is to maintain harmony in the use of animals, humans and material resources. Avoid delay in research and development of new drugs. Maintain the safeguards on safety, quality and efficacy along with regulatory obligations to protect public health.

1.4.3 Structure of ICH

ICH structurally made up of regulatory and industry as equal partners. It is a part of discussion both scientifically and technically for testing procedures to make sure regarding quality, safety and efficacy of medicines. ICH also focuses on the technical check of medicinal products containing potent drugs. Initially, ICH was confined to applicable only for three regions i.e. United States of America, Japan and Western Europe.

ICH is comprised of six parties that act as regulatory bodies; these parties include European Union (EU), European Federation of Pharmaceutical Industries Associations (EFPIA), Ministry of Health Labour and Welfare (MHLW), Japan Pharmaceutical Manufactures Association (JPMA), US Food and Drug Administrations (USFDA) and **Pharmaceutical Research and Manufacturers of America (Phrma)**

(a) European Union (EU)

EU is represented by the 27 members of European Commission that works for the harmonization of legislation along with technical necessities with the aim to achieve a single market in pharmaceuticals. It may help in free movement of products throughout the EU.

(b) European Federation of Pharmaceutical Industries Associations (EFPIA)

EFPIA deals in manufacturing, growth and research of medicinal products for human use in Europe. It is situated in Brussels and composed of 45 leading pharmaceutical companies and 29 national pharmaceutical industries.

(c) Ministry of Health, Labour and Welfare, Japan (MHLW)

MHLW plays the role of approval and administration of drugs, cosmetics and medical devices in Japan.

(d) Japan Pharmaceutical Manufacturers Association (JPMA)

JPMA is a major research based pharmaceutical manufacturers association in Japan. It is represented by 14 committees and 75 members that includes 20 foreign affiliates.

(e) US Food and Drug Administration (USFDA)

USFDA deals in wide range of responsibilities including drugs and cosmetics, medical devices, radiological and biological products. It gives approval for drugs and drug products in USA. It consists of regulatory, scientific and administrative committees that works under the office of Commissioner and other regulating centers. Center for

Biologics Evaluation and Research (CBER) and Center for Drug Evaluation and Research (CDER) are responsible for drawing technical advice to ICH.

(f) Pharmaceutical Research and Manufacturers of America (PhRMA)

PhRMA is a research-based industry in the USA that is associated with 67 companies involved in research, development and manufacturing of medicine along with 24 research affiliates that engaged in development of vaccines and drugs. Structure of ICH is shown in Figure 1.2 (a).

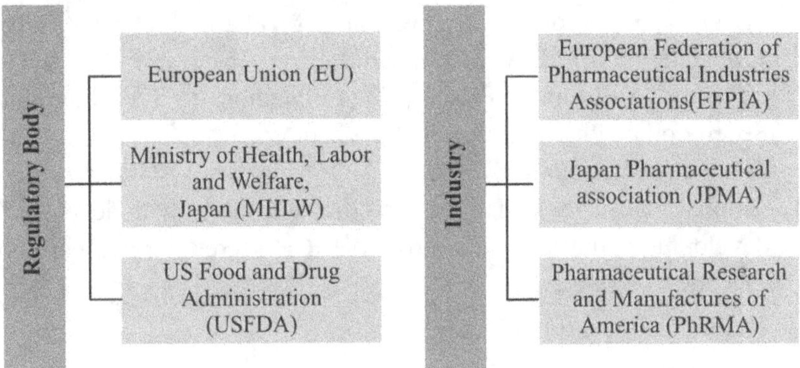

Figure 1.2 (a) Structure of ICH.

1.4.4 Purpose of ICH

- Harmonization of technical requirements
- Ensure safety, efficacy, and quality of medicines
- Avoidance of clinical trials duplication in humans
- Reduce number of animals in pre-clinical studies without compromising safety and effectiveness of the testing

1.4.5 Organization of ICH

The organization of ICH is shown in Figure 1.2 (b).

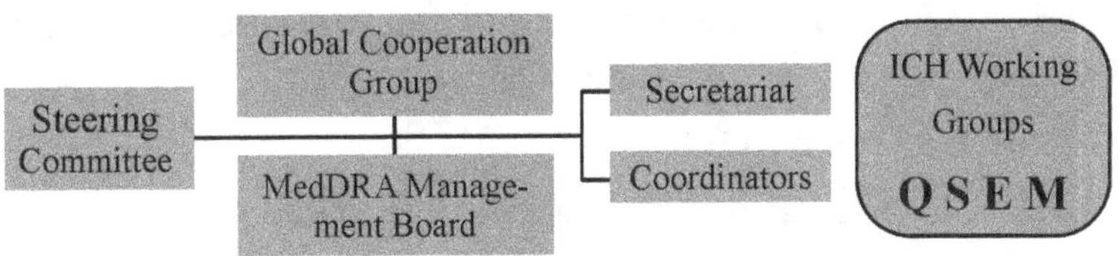

Where Med DRA = medical dictionary of regulatory activities, Q = quality, S = safety, E = efficacy, M = management

Figure 1.2 (b) Organization of ICH.

(a) Steering Committee (SC)

ICH is administered by the ICH Steering Committee which is supported by the ICH Secretariat. The Steering Committee, works with the ICH terms of reference, determines the policies and procedures for ICH, selects topics for harmonization and monitors the progress of harmonization initiatives. The steering committee meets at least twice a year with the location changing between the three regions. It has six co-sponsors that are European Union (EU), Ministry of Health, Labor and Welfare, Japan (MHLW), US Food and Drug Administration (US-FDA) and European Federation of Pharmaceutical Industries Associations (EFPIA). SC includes three observers; WHO, Health Canada and European Free Trade Association (EFTA). International Federation of Pharmaceutical Manufacturers & Associations (IFPMA) is a non-profit, non-governmental Organization (NGO) representing national industry associations and companies from both developed and developing countries which hosts the ICH secretariat and participates as a non-voting member.

(b) Global Cooperation Group

It is a subcommittee of SC formed in 1999.

(c) Med DRA management board

This board is responsible to observe the activities of the "Maintenance and Support Services Organization" (MSSO).

(d) Secretariat and Coordinators

Secretariat of SC is located in Geneva, Switzerland operating from International Federation of Pharmaceutical Manufacturers Associations (IFPMA) offices. Coordinators are the fundamental unit responsible for smooth running of ICH.

(e) ICH working groups

ICH working groups includes Implementation Working Group (IWG), Expert Working Group (EWG), Discussion Group and Informal Working Group. It can be divided into four categories QSEM followed by assigning ICH topic codes to these categories.

(f) Quality Guidelines (Q)

Quality can be evaluated by conduction of stability studies, testing of impurities and risk management based on Good Manufacturing Practice (GMP).

Table 1.1 List of quality guidelines

Q1 A	Stability Testing of New Drug Substances and Products
Q1 B	Stability Testing Photostability Testing of New Drug Substances and Products
Q1C	Stability Testing for New Dosage Forms
Q1D	Bracketing and Matrixing Designs for Stability Testing of New Drugs Substances and Products
Q1E	Evaluation for Stability Data
Q2	Validation of Analytical Procedures: Text and Methodology
Q3A	Impurities in New Drug Substances
Q3B	Impurities in New Drug Products
Q3C	Impurities: Guidelines for Residual Solvents
Q3D	Impurities: Guidelines for Elemental Impurities
Q4	Evaluation and Recommendation of Pharmacopoeial Texts for Use in the ICH Regions
Q5A	Viral safety Evaluation of Biotechnology Products Derived from Cell Lines of Human or Animal Origin
Q5B	Quality of Biotechnology Products: Production of rDNA Derived Protein Products
Q5C	Quality of Biotechnology Products: Stability Testing of Biotechnological/Biological Products
Q5D	Derivation and Characterization of Cell Substrates Used for Production of Biotechnological/Biological Products
Q5E	Comparability of Biotechnological/Biological Products Subject to Changes in their Manufacturing Process
Q6A	Specifications: Test Procedures and Acceptance Criteria for New Drug Substances and New Drug Products: Chemical Substances
Q6B	Specifications: Test Procedures and Acceptance Criteria for Biotechnological/Biological Products
Q7	Good Manufacturing Practice Guide for Active Pharmaceutical Ingredients
Q8	Pharmaceutical Development
Q9	Quality Risk Management
Q10	Pharmaceutical Quality System
Q11	Development and Manufacture of Drug Substances
Q12	Lifecycle management
Q13	Continuous manufacture of drug substances and drug products
Q14	Analytical procedure development

1.4.6 Safety Guidelines (S)

ICH has made complete set of safety guidelines, so as to minimize certain risks likes carcinogenicity, genotoxicity and reprotoxicity. A recent advancement has been a non-clinical testing strategy for assessing the QT interval prolongation liability: the single most important cause of drug withdrawals in recent years. List of safety guidelines is shown in Table 1.2.

Table 1.2 List of safety guidelines

S1A	Guidelines on the Need for Carcinogenicity Studies of Pharmaceuticals
S1B	Testing for Carcinogenicity of Pharmaceuticals
S1C	Dose Selection for Carcinogenicity Studies of Pharmaceuticals
S2	Guidance on Genotoxicity Testing and Data Interpretation for Pharmaceuticals Intended for Human Use
S3A	Note for Guidance on Toxicokinetics: The Assessment of Systemic Exposure in Toxicity Studies
S3B	Pharmacokinetics: Guidance for Repeated Dose Tissue Distribution Studies
S4	Duration of Chronic Toxicity Testing in Animals
S5	Detection of Toxicity to Reproduction for Medicinal Products and Toxicity to Male Fertility
S6	Preclinical Safety Evaluation of Biotechnology-Derived Pharmaceuticals
S7A	Safety Pharmacology Studies for Human Pharmaceuticals
S7B	Non-clinical Evaluation of the Potential for Delayed Ventricular Repolarization by Human Pharmaceuticals
S8	Immunotoxicity Studies for Human Pharmaceuticals
S9	Nonclinical Evaluation for Anticancer Pharmaceuticals
S10	Photosafety Evaluation

1.4.7 Efficacy Guidelines

The work carried out by ICH under the Efficacy heading is concerned with the design, conduct, and safety and reporting of clinical trials. It also covers novel types of medicines derived from biotechnological processes and the use of pharmacogenetics/genomics techniques to produce better targeted medicines. List of efficacy guidelines is shown in Table 1.3.

Table 1.3 List of efficacy guidelines

E1	The extent of populations Exposure to Assess Clinical Safety for Drugs Intended for Long-Term Treatment of Non -Life-Threatening Conditions
E2A	Clinical Safety Data Management: Definitions and Standards for Expedited Reporting
E2B	Clinical Safety Data Management: Data Elements for Transmission of Individual Case Safety Reports
E2C	Periodic Benefit-Risk Evaluation Report

Table 1.3 *Contd...*

E2D	Post-Approval Safety Data Management
E2E	Pharmacovigilance Planning
E2F	Development Safety Update Report
E3	Structure and Content of Clinical Study Reports
E4	Dose-Response Information to Support Drug Registration
E5	Ethnic Factors in the Acceptability of Foreign Clinical Data
E6	Good Clinical Practice: Consolidated Guideline
E7	Studies in Support of Special Populations: Geriatrics
E8	General Considerations for Clinical Trials
E9	Statistical Principles for Clinical Trials
E10	Choice of Control Group and Related Issues in Clinical Trials
E11	Clinical Investigation of Medicinal Products in the Pediatric Population
E12	Principles for Clinical Evaluation of New Anti hypretensive Drugs
E14	Clinical Evaluation of QT/QTc Interval Prolongation and Proarrhythmic Potential for Non-Ant arrhythmic Drugs
E15	Definitions for Genomic Biomarkers, Pharmacogenomics, Pharmacogenetics, Genomic Data and Sample Coding Categories
E16	Biomarkers Related to Drug or Biotechnology Product Development: Context, Structure and Format of Qualification Submissions

1.4.8 Multidisciplinary Guidelines

Those are the cross-cutting topics which do not fit uniquely into one of the Quality, Safety and Efficacy categories. It includes the ICH medical terminology, the Common Technical Document (CTD) and the development of Electronic Standards for the Transfer of Regulatory Information (ESTRI). List of multidisciplinary guidelines is shown in Table 1.4.

Table 1.4 D List of multidisciplinary guidelines

M1	MedDRA Terminology
M2	Electronic Transmission of Individual Case Safety Reports
M3	Guidance on Nonclinical Safety Studies for the Conduct of Human Clinical Trials and Marketing Authorization for Pharmaceuticals
M4	Organization of the Common Technical Document for the Registration of Pharmaceuticals for Human Use
M5	Data elements and standards for drug dictionaries
M6	Gene therapy
M7	Assessment and Control of DNA Reactive Impurities in Pharmaceuticals to Limit Potential Carcinogenic Risk

1.5 Organization for Economic Co-operation and Development (OECD)

Various chemicals such as pesticides, food additives, biotechnology products, industrial chemicals and pharmaceuticals arrive at the world marketplace every year. These chemicals need safety testing in most parts of the world. OECD in 1981in collaboration with its countries and its partners has developed various guidelines and these guidelines must be followed by everyone. It includes a number of advantages such as:

- It increases the validity, legality and international recognition of test data.

- Create the excellent use of existing resources in both governments and industry.

- Avoid the unnecessary use of laboratory animals.

- Decreases non-tariff trade barriers.

1.5.1 The OECD Test Guidelines

- It includes safety testing of chemicals. These testing should be in accordance with its physicochemical properties, effects on biotic systems (ecotoxicity), environmental fate properties, health effects (toxicity), and other areas such as pesticide residue chemistry and efficacy testing of biocides.

- These guidelines are internationally accepted as standard methods for safety testing and provide the common basis for the mutual acceptance of test data.

- These are essential for professionals working in industry, academia and government on the testing and assessment of chemical substances.

- Main aim is to reflect the current state-of-the-art in hazard identification and characterization testing.

- The guidelines are updated in order to keep pace with progress in science, and to address animal welfare concerns.

- The OECD accepted the need to protect animals in general and in particular those used in experimental work 25 years ago. These guidelines are followed throughout the world.

1.5.2 General Guidelines for Designing and Conducting Toxicity Studies

(a) Good Laboratory Practice

Nonclinical laboratory studies must be performed according to U.S. FDA good laboratory practice (GLP) regulations.

- **Care, maintenance and housing:** Recommendations about the care, maintenance, and housing of animals

- **Selection of species, strains and sex:** These guidelines are generally used for rodents (usually rats) and non-rodents (usually dogs). In case other species are used, modifications of these guidelines are necessary. Male and female test animals both can be used. Healthy animals (with no previous experiment) are chosen for experiments. It is necessary to think about the animal's sensitivity and the responsiveness of particular organs and tissues before performing any toxicity studies. One should be careful about rodent species, strains, and sub strains for toxicity studies.

- **Age:** Testing is usually done on young animals. These animals are acclimatized for at least 5 days, then only any experiment can be performed on them. Drug administration to rodents should begin no later than 6 to 8 weeks of age. When dogs are used, drug administration should begin no later than 4 to 6 months of age.

- **Number and sex:** Equal numbers of males and females of each species and strain should be used for the study. For sub chronic toxicity studies, experimental and control groups should have at least 20 rodents/sex/group or at least 4 dogs/sex/group. 10 rodents/sex/group may be suitable for sub chronic rodent studies when the study is considered to be range-finding in nature or when longer term studies are anticipated. These recommendations will assure that the number of animals that survive until the end of the study will be sufficient to permit significant evaluation of toxicological effects.

- **Infected animals:** Generally, it is not possible to treat animals for infection during the course of a study without risking interaction between the compound used for treatment and the test substance. This interaction may confound or complicate the interpretation of study results.

- **Animal identification:** Test animals should be characterized by reference to their species, strain (and sub strain), sex, age, and weight. Each animal must be assigned a unique identification number (e.g., ear tag, implanted identification chip, tattoo).
Caging: Animals should be housed one per cage or run (single-caged) except during mating and lactation and for acute toxicity studies. This recommendation reflects three points of consideration:

  (i) The amount of feed consumed by each animal in the study cannot be determined when more than one animal is housed in each cage. This information is necessary in the determination of feed efficiency (relationship of feed consumed to body weight gained).

(ii) Minimizing the possibility of confounding analyses and determining whether decreases in body weight gain are due to decreased palatability or substance mediated toxicity.

(iii) Organs and tissues from moribund and dead animals which are single-caged would not be lost due to cannibalism.

- **Diet:** In general, feed and water should be provided *ad libitum* to animals in toxicity studies, and the diets for these studies should meet the nutritional requirements of the species for normal growth and reproduction. Unless special circumstances apply which justify otherwise, care should be taken to ensure that the diets of the compound treated groups of animals are is caloric (equivalent in caloric density) with and contain the same levels of nutrients (e.g., fiber, micronutrients) as the diets of the control group. Unrecognized or inadequately controlled dietary variables may result in nutritional imbalances or caloric deprivation that could confound interpretation of the toxicity study results (e.g., lifespan, background rates of tumor incidences) and alter the outcome and reproducibility of the studies.

1.5.3 Assignment of Control and Compound Treated Animals

Animals should be assigned to control and compound treated groups in a stratified random manner. Animals in all groups should be placed on study on the same day; if this is not possible because of the large number of animals in a study, animals may be placed on study over several days. If the latter recommendation is followed, a preselected portion of the control and experimental animals should be placed on the study each day in order to maintain concurrence.

- **Mortality:** Excessive mortality due to poor animal management is unacceptable and may cause to repeat the study. For example, under normal circumstances, mortality in the control group should not exceed 10% in short and intermediate length (not lifetime) toxicity studies.

- **Autolysis:** Adequate animal husbandry practices should result in considerably less than 10% of animals and tissues or organs lost to a study because of autolysis. Autolysis in excess of this standard may result in repetition of the study.

- **Necropsy:** If the animal is found dead or sacrificed after the experiment then necropsy should be performed immediately to avoid the autolysis. When necropsy cannot be performed immediately, the animal should be refrigerated at a low temperature but temperature should not be so low so it can cause tissue damage. If histopathological examination is necessary then tissue specimens should be taken from the animals and placed in appropriate fixatives.

1.5.4 Test Substance

The test substance should be the same that the petitioner should market. The toxicity study of the substance should be carried out. A single batch of test substance should be used throughout the study, when possible. Alternatively, batch that is as similar as possible in purity and composition should be used.

- **Identity:** The identity of the test substance or mixture of substances to be tested should be known. Petitioners should consult with the Agency in determination of test compound and to provide a Chemical Abstract Service (CAS) Registry Number or Numbers.

- **Composition/purity:** The composition of the test substance should be known including the name and quantities of all major components, known contaminants and impurities, and the percentage of unidentifiable materials.

- **Conditions of storage:** The test sample should be kept under conditions that preserve its firmness, quality, and cleanliness till the studies are going on.

- **Expiration date:** The expiration date of the test material should be well known. Test materials should not be used after the expiry date.

1.5.5 Experimental Design

- **Duration of testing:** Animals should be exposed to the test substance 7 days per week for the designated time of the study.

- **Route of administration:** The route of administration of the test substance should match with that of same route used for human if it is possible. For food ingredients (e.g., food and color additives) the oral route of administration is preferred. Proper justification should be provided when other routes are used. The same method of administration should be used for all test animals throughout the study. The test substance should be administered in one of the following ways:

  (i) In the diet: If human should take the test substance through solid food or a mixture of solid and liquid food, test substance is mixed with the diet. Animals should take the diet completely so that complete dose of the test substance is taken by the animals. If the test substance is added with ground feed, the test substance should not lose its basic properties during or after pelleting. When the test substance is administered in the diet, dietary levels should be expressed as mg of the test substance per kg of feed.

(ii) Dissolved in the drinking water: Test substance is given through liquid form when it cannot be given through diet. It is given along with water or with some suitable solvents. The amount of test substance administered in drinking water should be expressed as mg of test substance per ml of water.

(iii) By encapsulation or oral intubation: If the two previous methods are not suitable or the animals require large dose then the animal should be given dose by oral gavage. If the test substance is administered by gavage, it should be given at exact the same dose each time a day. The maximum volume of solution that can be given by gavage in one dose depends on the size of animal. For rodents, the volume ordinarily should not exceed 1 ml/100 g body weight. If the gavage vehicle is oil, then the volume should be not more than 0.4 ml/100 g of body weight. If the test substance must be given in divided doses, all doses should be administered within a 6 hour period. Doses of test substance administered by gavage should be expressed as mg of test substance per ml of gavage vehicle.

- **Dose groups:** Three to five dose levels of the test substance and concurrent control groups should be used with both males and females. Information obtained from acute and short-term toxicity studies can help determine appropriate doses for sub chronic studies.

- **Selection of treatment doses:** Dose is appropriately selected for toxicity studies. It should depend on information related to the toxicity of the test substance. A minimum of three dose levels of the test substance and a concurrent control group should be used in toxicity studies. While performing toxicity studies various factors should be considered:

    (i) The high dose should be adequately high to induce toxic responses in test animals.

    (ii) The low dose should not induce toxic responses in test animals.

    (iii) The intermediate dose should be sufficiently high to elicit minimal toxic effects in test animals (such as alterations in enzyme levels or slight decreases in body weight gains).

    (iv) No dose should cause an incidence of fatalities that prevents meaningful evaluation of the data. Administration of the test substance to all dose groups should be done concurrently.

- **Controls:** A concurrent control group of test animals is required. The control group in dietary studies should be fed the basal diet. A carrier or vehicle for the test substance should be given to control animals at a volume equal to the maximum volume of carrier or vehicle given to any dosed group of animals.

1.5.6 Computerized Systems

Computerized systems that are used in the generation, measurement, or assessment of data should be developed, validated, operated, and maintained in ways that are compliant with Good Laboratory Practice principles.

1.5.7 Observations and Clinical Tests

(a) **Observations of Test Animals:** Routine cage-side observations should be made on all animals at least once or twice a day throughout the study for general signs of pharmacologic and toxicologic effects, morbidity and mortality. The usual interval between observations should be at least 6 hours. Individual records should be maintained for each animal and the time of onset and the uniqueness and progression of any effects should be recorded, preferably using a scoring system. An expanded set of clinical evaluations, performed inside and outside of the cage, should be carried out in short-term and subchronic toxicity studies in rodents and non-rodents, in one-year non-rodent toxicity studies, and reproductive toxicity studies in rodents to enable detection not only of general pharmacologic and toxicologic effects but also of neurologic disorders, behavioral changes, autonomic dysfunctions, and other signs of nervous system toxicity. Signs noted should include, but not be limited to, changes in skin, fur, eyes, and mucous membranes, occurrence of secretions and excretions and autonomic activity (e.g., lacrimation, piloerection, pupil size, and unusual respiratory pattern). Additionally, changes in gait, posture and response to handling, as well as the presence of clonic or tonic movements, stereotypes (e.g., excessive grooming, repetitive circling) or bizarre behavior (e.g., self-mutilating, walking backwards) should be recorded. Tumor development, particularly in long-term studies, should be followed: the time of onset, location, dimensions, appearance and progression of each grossly visible or palpable tumor should be recorded. During the course of a study, toxic and pharmacologic signs may suggest the need for supplementary clinical tests or expanded post-mortem examinations.

(b) **Body Weight and Feed Intake Data:** Feed spillage should be noted and adjustments made in related calculations.

(c) **Clinical Testing:** Ophthalmological examination, hematology profiles, clinical chemistry tests, and urinalyses are few clinical tests that should be performed as described in the following sections

(d) **Ophthalmological Examination:** This examination should be performed by a qualified individual on all animals before the study begins and on control and high-dose animals at the end of the study. If the results of examinations at termination indicate that changes in the eyes may be associated with administration of the test substance, ophthalmological examinations should be performed on all animals in the study.

(e) Hematology: Blood samples should be analyzed individually, and not pooled. If animals are sampled on more than one day during a study, blood should be drawn at approximately the same time each sampling day. The following determinations are recommended:

- Hematocrit
- Hemoglobin concentration
- Erythrocyte count
- Total and differential leukocyte counts
- Mean corpuscular hemoglobin
- Mean corpuscular volume
- Mean corpuscular hemoglobin concentration
- Measurement of clotting potential (such as clotting time, prothrombin time, thromboplastin time, or platelet count)

  Test compounds may produce effect on the hematopoietic system. Therefore suitable actions should be performed for evaluations of reticulocyte counts and bone marrow cytology. Reticulocyte counts should be attained for each animal using automated reticulocyte counting capabilities, or from air-dried blood smears. Bone marrow slides should be prepared from each animal for evaluating bone marrow cytology. These slides would only need to be examined microscopically if effects on the hematopoietic system were noted.

(f) Clinical Chemistry: Blood samples should be drawn at the end of the fasting time and before feeding. Fasting duration should be appropriate for the species and the analytical tests to be performed. Clinical chemistry tests that are appropriate for all test substances include measurements of electrolyte balance, carbohydrate metabolism, and liver and kidney function. Specific determinations should include:

(i) Hepatocellular evaluation: select at least 3 of the following 5 parameters

- Alanine aminotransferase (SGPT, ALT)
- Aspartate aminotransferase (SGOT, AST)
- Sorbitol dehydrogenase (SDH)
- Glutamate dehydrogenase
- Total bile acids

(ii) Hepatobiliary evaluation: select at least 3 of the following 5

- Alkaline phosphatase (ALP)

- Bilirubin (total)
- Gamma-glutamyltranspeptidase (GG transferase)
- 5' nucleotidase
- Total bile acids

(iii) Other markers of cell changes or cellular function

- Albumin
- Calcium chloride
- Total cholesterol
- Cholinesterase
- Creatinine
- Globulin
- Glucose (in fasted animals)
- Phosphorous
- Potassium
- Total Protein
- Sodium triglycerides
- Urea

(g) Urinalyses: Timed urine volume collection should be conducted during the last week of the study. The volume of urine collected, specific gravity, pH, glucose, and protein should be determined as well as conducting a microscopic evaluation of urine for sediment and presence of blood/blood cells.

(h) Neurotoxicity Screening/Testing: Screening for neurotoxic effects should be routinely carried out in short-term and subchronic toxicity studies with rodents (preferably rats) and non-rodents (preferably dogs), one-year studies in non-rodents, and reproductive toxicity studies in rodents.

(i) Immunotoxicity: For short-term, subchronic and developmental toxicity studies, results of clinical tests that are included in the list of primary indicators for immune toxicity should also be evaluated as part of an immunotoxicity screen. Additional immunotoxicity tests.

(j) Necropsy and microscopic Examination Gross necropsy: All test animals should be subjected to complete gross necropsy, including examination of external surfaces, orifices, cranial, thoracic and abdominal cavities, carcass, and all other organs. The gross necropsy should be performed by, or under the direct supervision of, a qualified pathologist, preferably the person who will later perform the microscopic examination.

(k) Organ weight: Organs like adrenals, brain, epididymis, heart, kidneys, liver, spleen, testes, thyroid/parathyroid, thymus, ovaries and uterus should be weighed. Organs should be carefully dissected and trimmed to remove fat and other contagious tissue and then be weighed immediately to minimize the effects of drying on weight of organ.

(l) Preparation of Tissues for Microscopic Examination Generally, the following tissues should be fixed in 10% buffered formalin (or another generally recognized fixative) and sections prepared and stained with hematoxylin and eosin (or another appropriate stain) in preparation for microscopic examination. Lungs should be inflated with fixative prior to immersion in fixative.

(m) Microscopic Evaluation: All gross lesions should be examined microscopically. All tissues from the animals in the control and high dose groups should be examined. If treatment related effects are noted in certain tissues, then the next lower dose level tested of those specific tissues should be examined. Successive examination of the next lower dose level continues until no effects are noted. In addition, all tissues from animals which died prematurely or were sacrificed during the study should be examined microscopically to assess any potential toxic effects.

(n) Histopathology of Lymphoid Organs: Histopathological evaluation of the lymphoid organs should be performed for all animals in short-term and sub chronic toxicity studies and developmental toxicity studies. Different OECD guidelines for testing of chemicals is shown in Table 1.5.

Table 1.5 Different OECD guidelines for testing of chemicals

Test No. 401	Acute Oral Toxicity
Test No. 402	Acute Dermal Toxicity
Test No. 403	Acute Inhalation Toxicity
Test No. 404	Acute Dermal Irritation/Corrosion
Test No. 405	Acute Eye Irritation/Corrosion
Test No. 406	Skin Sensitisation
Test No. 407	Repeated Dose 28-day Oral Toxicity Study in Rodents
Test No. 408	Repeated Dose 90-Day Oral Toxicity Study in Rodents
Test No. 409	Repeated Dose 90-Day Oral Toxicity Study in Non-Rodents
Test No. 410	Repeated Dose Dermal Toxicity: 21/28-day Study
Test No. 411	Subchronic Dermal Toxicity: 90-day Study
Test No. 412	Repeated Dose Inhalation Toxicity: 28-day or 14-day Study
Test No. 413	Subchronic Inhalation Toxicity: 90-day Study

Table 1.5 *Contd...*

Test No. 414	Prenatal Development Toxicity Study
Test No. 415	One-Generation Reproduction Toxicity Study
Test No. 416	Two-Generation Reproduction Toxicity
Test No. 417	Toxicokinetics
Test No. 418	Delayed Neurotoxicity of Organophosphorus Substances
Test No. 419	Delayed Neurotoxicity of Organophosphorus Substances: 28-day
Test No. 420	Acute Oral Toxicity - Fixed Dose Procedure
Test No. 421	Reproduction/Developmental Toxicity Screening Test
Test No. 422	Combined Repeated Dose Toxicity Study with the Reproduction/Developmental Toxicity Screening Test
Test No. 423	Acute Oral toxicity - Acute Toxic Class Method
Test No. 424	Neurotoxicity Study in Rodents
Test No. 425	Acute Oral Toxicity: Up-and-Down Procedure
Test No. 426	Developmental Neurotoxicity Study
Test No. 427	Skin Absorption: In Vivo Method
Test No. 428	Skin Absorption: *In vitro* Method
Test No. 429	Skin Sensitisation: Local Lymph Node Assay
Test No. 430	*In vitro* Skin Corrosion: Transcutaneous Electrical Resistance Test (TER)
Test No. 431	*In vitro* Skin Corrosion: Human Skin Model Test
Test No. 432	*In vitro* 3T3 NRU Phototoxicity Test
Test No. 435	*In vitro* Membrane Barrier Test Method for Skin Corrosion
Test No. 440	Uterotrophic Bioassay in Rodents: A short-term screening test for oestrogenic properties
Test No. 451	Carcinogenicity Studies
Test No. 452	Chronic Toxicity Studies
Test No. 453	Combined Chronic Toxicity/Carcinogenicity Studies
Test No. 471	Bacterial Reverse Mutation Test
Test No. 473	*In vitro* Mammalian Chromosome Aberration Test
Test No. 474	Mammalian Erythrocyte Micronucleus Test
Test No. 475	Mammalian Bone Marrow Chromosome Aberration Test
Test No. 476	*In vitro* Mammalian Cell Gene Mutation Test
Test No. 482	Genetic Toxicology: DNA Damage and Repair, Unscheduled DNA Synthesis in Mammalian Cells *in vitro*
Test No. 483	Mammalian Spermatogonial Chromosome Aberration Test
Test No. 484	Genetic Toxicology: Mouse Spot Test
Test No. 485	Genetic toxicology, Mouse Heritable Translocation Assay
Test No. 486	Unscheduled DNA Synthesis (UDS) Test with Mammalian Liver Cells *in vivo*

1.6   United States Food and Drug Administration (USFDA)

The USFDA is an organization of Department of Health and Human Services (HHS) in United States. This body is responsible for due care of the public health by assuring the protection, effectiveness, and security of human and veterinary drugs, vaccines and other biological products, medical devices, national food supply, cosmetics, dietary supplements, and products that give off radiation. In order for drugs, medical devices, and other products to be approved, the FDA does not require that animals be used in product testing and drug development. Instead, it requires that certain safety and efficacy tests be met and as such has the authority to vastly reduce the number of animal tests by making the use of existing, validated alternatives mandatory.

1.6.1 FDA Fundamentals

The Food and Drug Administration (FDA) is an agency within the U.S. Department of Health and Human Services. It comprises of the Office of the Commissioner and four directorates overseeing the core functions of the agency: Medical Products and Tobacco, Foods and Veterinary Medicine, Global Regulatory Operations and Policy, and Operations.

1.6.2 Office of the Commissioner

The office collectively performs leadership of the agency's scientific activities, communication, legislative liaison, policy and planning, women's and minority health initiatives, agency operations, and toxicological research.

1.6.3 Office of Foods and Veterinary Medicine

This office addresses food and feed safety, nutrition, and other critical areas to achieve public health goals.

1.6.4 Office of Global Regulatory Operations and Policy

It provides leadership for FDA's domestic and international product quality and safety efforts.

1.6.5 Office of Medical Products and Tobacco

Advice and counsel to the Commissioner on all medical product and tobacco-related programs and issues.

1.6.6 Office of Operations

It provides agency-wide services including information technology, financial management, procurement, library services, and freedom of information, FDA history, and facilities.

1.6.7 Responsibilities of FDA

FDA is responsible for protecting the public health by assuring the safety, effectiveness, quality, and security of human and veterinary drugs, vaccines and other biological products, and medical devices. The FDA is also responsible for the safety and security of most of nation's food supply, all cosmetics, dietary supplements and products that produce any kind of radiation.

- It protects the public from electronic product radiation.
- It ensures that cosmetics and dietary supplements are safe and properly labeled
- It regulates tobacco products.
- It progress the public health by increasing product innovations.

1.6.8 FDA Structure/ Organization: Structure of FDA is Depicted in Figure 1.3 (a)

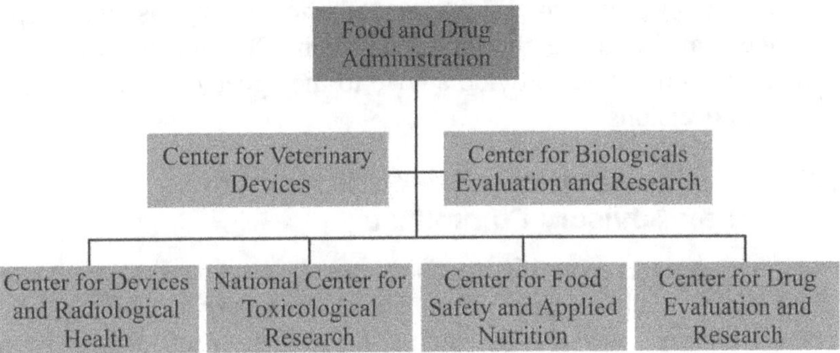

Figure 1.3 (a) Structure of FDA.

1.6.9 Scope of FDA

The scope of FDA's regulatory authority is very broad. The following is a list of traditionally-recognized product categories that fall under FDA's regulatory jurisdiction; In general, FDA regulates:

- Foods, including: dietary supplements, bottled water, food additives, infant formulas
- Drugs, including: prescription drugs (both brand-name and generic), non-prescription (over-the-counter) drugs

- Biologics, including: vaccines, blood and blood products, cellular and gene therapy products, tissue and tissue products, allergenic

- Medical Devices, including: tongue depressors and bedpans, complex technologies such as heart pacemakers, dental devices, surgical implants and prosthetics

- Electronic Products that give off radiation, including: microwave ovens, x-ray equipment, laser products, ultrasonic therapy equipment, mercury vapor lamps, sunlamps

- Cosmetics, including: color additives found in makeup and other personal care products, skin moisturizers and cleansers, nail polish and perfume

- Veterinary Products, including: livestock feeds, pet foods, veterinary drugs and devices

- Tobacco Products, including: cigarettes, cigarette tobacco, roll-your-own tobacco, smokeless tobacco

1.6.10 FDA Advisory Committee

FDA has an advisory committee. It provides special advices on problems related to human and veterinary drugs, vaccines and other biological products, medical devices, and food. In general, advisory committees include a chairperson, several members, a consumer, industry, and sometimes a patient representative. Additional experts with special knowledge may be added for individual committee meetings as needed. Although the committees provide advice to the agency, FDA has the right to take final decisions.

1.6.11 Qualifications of a Scientific Member of an Advisory Committee

Persons suggested as scientific members must be technically skilled experts in their field, such as clinical medicine, engineering, biological and physical sciences, biostatistics and food sciences. They also must have knowledge about interpretation and analysis of all scientific data, and understanding its public health significance.

1.7   Necessity of Animals for Testing of Medical Products

For testing of drugs, vaccines and other biologics, and medical devices animals are used to determine the safety of the medical product.

For drugs and biologics, the focus of animal testing is on the drug's nature, chemistry, and effects (pharmacology) and on its potential damage to the body (toxicology). Animal testing is used to measure:

- What is the bioavailability of the drug or biologics?
- What is the pharmacokinetics of the drug or biologics?
- What is toxicity of the drug and its metabolites?
- What is the excretion rate of the product?

Medical devices need biocompatibility test before using on human body because it must be biocompatible with the human tissues. Most of the devices are made of materials stainless steel or ceramic that is biocompatible with human tissues, in these cases, no animal testing is required. However, some devices with novel materials require biocompatibility testing in animals.

There are still many areas where animal testing is essential. But FDA decreases the need of animal testing. FDA has been performing various research and development efforts which reduce the need for animal testing and to work toward replacement of animal testing.

1.8   Public Health Service Policy on Humane Care and Use of Laboratory Animals

The Public Health Service Policy on Humane Care and Use of Laboratory Animals (PHS Policy) was given in 1973 and revised in 1979 and 1986. The PHS Policy (NIH, 1986) applies to all institutions that use live vertebrates in research supported by any component of PHS: the Agency for Health Care Research and Quality, the Centers for Disease Control and Prevention, the Food and Drug Administration, the Health Resources and Services Administration, the Indian Health Service, the National Institutes of Health (NIH), and the Substance Abuse and Mental Health Services Administration. The PHS Policy requires institutions to establish and maintain proper measures to ensure the appropriate care and use of animals involved in research, research training, and biologic testing activities.

1.9 US Government Principles for the Utilization and Care of Vertebrate Animals used in Testing, Research and Training

The US Government Principles for the Utilization and Care of Vertebrate Animals Used in Testing, Research, and Training (US Government Principles) were drafted in 1985 by the Interagency Research Animal Committee (IRAC, 1985), made up of individuals drawn from federal agencies that use or require the use of animals in research or testing. Its nine statements address compliance with the animal welfare act (AWA) and other applicable federal laws, guidelines, and policies (such as AWRs, HREA, and the Guide) and generally provide a set of overarching principles for ensuring that the use of research animals is justified and humane.

1.10 Animal Welfare Act (AWA)

The Animal Welfare Act works in U.S. This Act is mainly for wellbeing of animals in research. The Act came into force in 1966. It regulates the care and use of animals in research, testing, teaching, exhibition, transport. AWA offer least protection for certain species while excluding others such as rats, mice, and birds. It does not apply to cold-blooded animals (fish, reptiles, and amphibians). This law applies to dogs, cats, nonhuman primates, guinea pigs, hamsters, rabbits. The law makes least standard for veterinary care, handling, feeding, and housing. It also maintains the psychological well being. Various government statistics gives approximate details that U.S. labs utilize 25 millions animals in a year. U.S. labs make use of 100 million genetically engineered animals.

1.11 The U.S. Department of Agriculture (USDA)

AWA is enforced by the U.S. Department of Agriculture (USDA). A animal Care program, Animal and Plant Health Inspection Service (APHIS) administers AWA regulations and standards.

Under the AWA, businesses and individuals using regulated animals must be licensed or registered with the USDA and facilities with regulated animals must be inspected yearly by APHIS. There is no legal requirement for the inspection of federally-owned and operated research facilities. The USDA has no jurisdiction over facilities using animals not covered under the AWA.

1.12 Institutional Animal Care and
Use Committee (IACUC)

Institutions or research organizations can establish an Institutional Animal Care and Use Committee (IACUC) under the AWA for monitoring and evaluation of the institution's animal care and use program. The responsibilities of IACUC's include:

- To check the facility providing for animal care and use program,
- To conduct inspection of the animal labs at least twice a year,
- To review and approve, disapprove, or modifications required in the research protocols.

- To respond, investigate and act on public complaints on animal care and use.
- To report about any shortcoming of animal care and use.
- To submit reports about the animal care and use to institution.

The IACUC is comprised of three members and including a veterinarian from the facility and one person not affiliated with the facility who will "provide representation for general community interests in the proper care and treatment of animals."

1.13 Association for Assessment and Accreditation of Laboratory Animal Care International (AAALAC)

Association for Assessment and Accreditation of Laboratory Animal Care International (AAALAC) is accreditation body to increase availability for government funding to the institutes or organization. It is a privately funded organization based on nonprofit membership that is financial supported from institutions it credits and inspects. It promotes humane care of animals. The aim of AAALAC is monitor and ensure the improvement and protection of the animals used in biomedical research. It follows the guidelines recommended for the Care and Use of Laboratory Animals. It is a self-policing association for accreditation.

References

- Shruthi, N. K., et.al. USFDA Guidelines on process validation - A Review. Int J Pharmtech Res.2014; 6 (3): 920-923.
- http://www.fda.gov/Drugs/GuidanceComplianceRegulatoryInformation/Guidances/default.htm
- http://www.neavs.org/research/laws
- https://www.fda.gov/Food/GuidanceRegulation/GuidanceDocumentsRegulatoryInformation/IngredientsAdditivesGRASPackaging/ucm078315.htm
- http://cpcsea.nic.in/Content/55_1_GUIDELINES.aspx
- https://www.meddra.org/about-meddra/organisation/management-board/phrma
- http://pharmaquest.weebly.com/uploads/9/9/4/2/9942916/10.pdf
- https://ntp.niehs.nih.gov/iccvam/suppdocs/feddocs/oecd/oecd_gl420.pdf
- http://www.oecd.org/env/ehs/testing/more-about-oecd-test-guidelines.htm

Chapter 2

Pharmacological Techniques for Evaluation of Drugs on Different Systems

2.1 Introduction

The techniques which are used to establish or to test/screen the therapeutic activity of test compound are termed as pharmacological screening techniques. Drug screening involves the sequence of experimentation and characterization for a leading molecule with a capacity to become a drug. The screening always involves various tests and it is believed that results of the test may permit the detection of physiological and pharmacological activity. The testing of synthetic organic compounds and of natural compound is being performed on a wide scale. Testing is generally done in pharmacological laboratories. The research departments of pharmaceutical based companies are always involved in searching new and potent pharmaceuticals.

The therapeutic and pharmacological approach generally decides the type and number of leading molecules for initial screening test. The mechanism and selectivity of the drug is also determined for better acceptance in the market. The toxic effects, if any present in the leading molecule may also revealed by screening the drug. However, undesired therapeutic action is suddenly discovered by the researcher. Various animal models are available depending upon the biological activity for selection of molecules. Good predictive preclinical models exist (for e.g., antibacterial, diabetes, renal performance, hypertension, thrombotic disease etc). For certain diseases like Alzheimer's disease there are very less pre-clinical animal models available for experimentation.

The major objective of screening is to determine that whether new substances are worthy or not for further experiment and to indicate which among them have the prominent therapeutic activities. There are three kinds of screening programs:

- **Single test** (screen for particular activity): The simple method to find substances that are active in a single way. For example hypoglycemic test which measures the ability of a compound to reduce the concentration of glucose in the blood.

- **Programmed test** (pharmacological effects): The test is based on evaluation of compounds for its activity. In this test the comparison study is performed between test and known compounds to predict the activity of the test compound. It also provides indications of potential side effects.

- **Blind test** (potential activities): This test is performed to determine the biological activity of new compounds in a group and find new areas of research. Since no activity of a definite type is anticipated, the program will evolve as the experience of the investigator increases.

2.2   Standardization of Drug

Bioassay is determination of potency of a substance and it is a great tool for screening and standardization of the drugs.

2.2.1 Principles of Bioassay

- To determine the potency of test compound by comparing it with the known or standard product under identical experimental conditions.

- The active compound should be known in both standard and test preparations.

- The assay should be designed in such a way that the effect is not similar as the desired therapeutic effect.

2.2.2 Pharmacological Applications of Bioassay

- To determine the potency of drugs

- Screening of the compounds obtained from natural source or synthetic compounds and their biological activities

- To establish SAR (structure activity relationship)

- For monitoring over environmental pollutants

- To determine pharmacological activities of new leading molecule

- To determine therapeutic advantage of a drug in comparison to other drug

- Bioassays are useful in study new leading compounds or other chemically mediated control systems

2.2.3 Standards

Standards are known and internationally accepted samples of drugs that is recommended by the Expert Committee of the Biological Standardization of World Health Organization (WHO). Normal drug response curve (DRC) is shown in Figure 2.1. From drug response curve we can compare the potency of unknown with the standard.

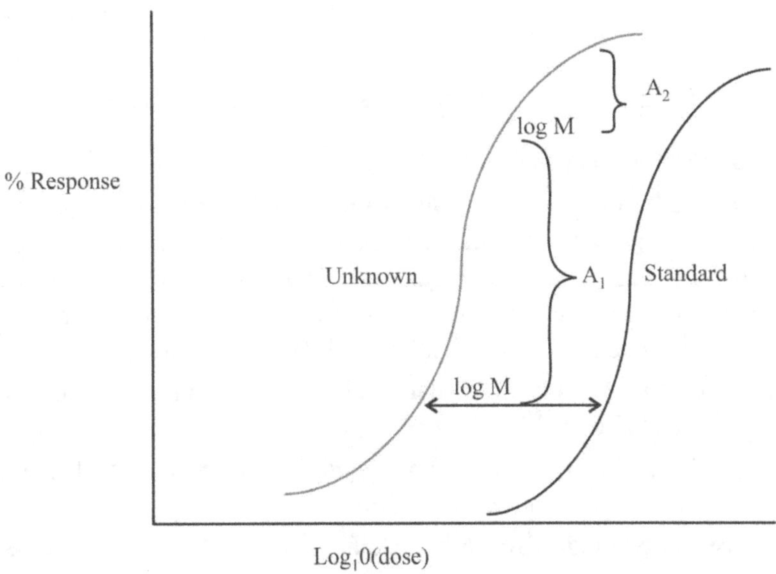

Figure 2.1 Comparitive study of potency of known and unknown compound by bioassay.

In this figure there is the comparison of response magnitude between known and unknown compounds. A_1 and A_2, are the differences chosen depending upon the dose. The comparative study provide a valid measure of relative potencies. The parallel lines show the magnitude of the effect; log M is the same at all points on the curves.

2.2.4 Dose-Response

Dose–response curve best defines the comparisons between the groups:

(a) Graded dose response: As the dose of the drug increases, response also increases in proportion. e.g. Insulin, as the dose is increased hypoglycemia increases. Graded dose response curve is shown in Figure 2.2.

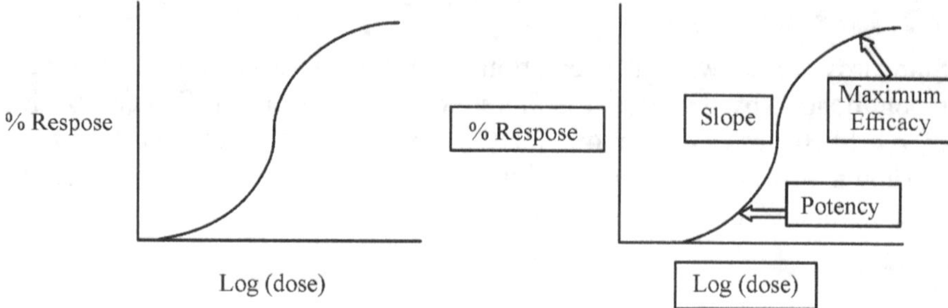

Figure 2.2 Basic characteristics of graded response.

(b) Quantal dose response

A quantal dose response is also called as all-or-none principal. In this response either there will be response or there will be no response. Dose-response relationship can be defined as the change in effect on an organism due to exposure of different doses of drug after a certain period of time e.g. effect of poison will be death or no death.

- **Molecular level:** Molecular level studies reveals about the receptor based studies.

- **Cellular level:** Cellular level study determines about the agonist and antagonist for a specific drug.

- **Systems/ Organism levels:** Animal study tells about the effect of drug on the whole animal body for e.g. effect of respiratory rates on dog.

There are several biological assays available at cellular, molecular, and whole animal levels for defining the activity and selectivity of the drug. Various pharmacological profile tests are shown in Table 2.1 A.

Table 2.1 Pharmacologic profile tests

Method of experiment	Species or Tissue	Measurement
Molecular level		
Binding with receptor (example: β-adrenoceptors)	Fractions of cell membrane from organs or cultured cells; cloned receptors	Affinity and selectivity of the receptor
Cytochrome P450	Liver	Enzyme inhibition; effects on drug metabolism
Enzymatic activity like dopamine-3-hydroxylase, tyrosine hydroxylase, monoamine oxidase	Adrenal glands; Sympathetic nerves; purified enzymes	Inhibition and selectivity of enzyme

Table 2.1 *Contd...*

Cellular level		
Cell function	Cultured cells	Activity of receptor – agonist or antagonist (example: effects on cyclic nucleotides)
Isolated tissue	Heart, blood vessels, , ileum (rat or guinea pig), lung	Effects on smooth muscles, contraction and relaxation on vascular system, selectivity for vascular receptors
Systems/Disease models		
Blood pressure	Dog, cat (anesthetized)	Systolic-diastolic changes
Cardiac effects	Dog (anesthetized)	Chronotropic and ionotropic effects, total peripheral resistance and cardiac output
Autonomic nervous system	Dog (anesthetized)	Effect of drug on stimulation of peripheral and central autonomic nervous system
Respiratory effects	Dog, guinea pig	Effects on bronchial tone, respiratory rate and amplitude
Diuretic activity	Dog	Renal blood flow, kaliuresis, natriuresis, glomerular filtration rate, water diuresis
Gastrointestinal effects	Rat	Gastrointestinal secretions and motility
Circulating hormones, cholesterol, blood sugar	Rat, dog	Serum concentration
Blood coagulation	Rabbit	Prothrombin time, clot retraction, coagulation time
Central nervous system	Mouse, rat	Muscle relaxation, locomotor activity, degree of sedation, stimulation

2.2.5 After Screening Via Bioassay

If the bioassay results are satisfactory, then there is a need for further chemical alterations so that bioavailability can be increased. For example:

- Administration of drugs through oral route may suggest about metabolism of the drugs and factors affecting bioavailability.

- Tolerance studies must be performed for drugs to be administered for longer time.
- The drugs which can produce dependence, various studies must be performed to know about the drug abuse potential.

2.2.6 Lead Compound

Lead compound is screened from various studies is the most active compound which can show pharmacological action. Lead compound is an important candidate for screening new drug.

2.2.7 Factors Affecting Pharmacological Response of Drugs

- **Sex:** The response of drug is different because of the different levels of metabolizing enzymes in both the sexes.
- **Age:** Along with age the metabolizing enzyme level also varies, however newborns lack in some enzymes.
- **Diseases:** Diseased condition may affect the pharmacological response of the drug e.g. kidney and liver disease.
- **Environmental:** Such as temperature, seasons, nutrition, light and isolation of animal etc. e.g. insulin produces convulsive action which is greatly affected by temperature.

2.2.8 Criteria of a Good Biological Assay

- **Selectivity:** Specific drug have affinity for specific receptor e.g. cholinergic drug will bind only with cholinergic system. In brief it can be concluded that signal transduction system is specific for specific drug.
- **Sensitivity:** Animal and their tissues give response to very less amount of drug and they are specific for their transduction system. (e.g. in histamine assay study, guinea pig ileum is more preferred because of presence of large amount of histaminase enzyme.)
- **Accuracy:** It can be defined as measurement of quantity to its true value.
- **Precision:** Precision is the degree that defines occurrence of same results under unchanged conditions of every measurement.

2.3   Pharmacological Approaches of Modern Medicine

Effect of drugs action on animals were first investigated by Rudolf Buchheim and Oswald Schmiedeberg in 19th century. Thus, pre-clinical studies started for the pharmacological evaluation of lead compounds. This is the reason that several drugs were discovered during the 20th century.

Conventional approach in pharmacological screening starts with testing of new chemical compound or new extracted biological compound on isolated animals followed by testing on whole animals such as in rats and mice. After pharmacological screening technique in the mid-1970s receptor binding studies came into existence for e.g. radioligand binding assay; and it has increased designing new chemical entities. Drug receptor technology also allows accelerated technique for interaction of small amount of compounds directly with the receptor or enzyme independently to its efficacy. Receptor pharmacology needs material and time for more division of receptors into various subclasses. In the search of novel agonists and antagonists, ligand binding assay has been proved as a potential tool along with identification of new classes of known receptors.

The conventional approach has the advantage of relatively high pertinence. The activity of antihypertensive compounds in rats is lower than humans. Dose response curve studies tell about the pharmacokinetic parameters and very little information is provided about their molecular mechanism but these approaches are time consuming and requires huge amount of compound. Additionally, this approach also provides little information about the molecular mechanisms involved in the observed effects, but one of the greatest achievements is that diabetes was treated with sulfonylureas since many years without knowing the exact mechanism.

2.4 New Approaches in Drug Discovery

2.4.1 Combinatorial Chemistry

Combinatorial chemistry is regular and repetitive covalent correlation including different set of 'building blocks' of varying structures to each other for providing a large collection of varied molecular entities. This branch of chemistry has become very popular but it is very tedious to make lead compound by scaffolding and to target the right signal transduction system.

2.4.2 High Throughput Screening

Development of receptor technology is carried out through high throughput screening. Various compounds are produced by combinatorial chemistry and their test can be performed in short period of time with high throughput screening.

2.4.3 Pharmacogenomics

Friedrich Vogel had coined the term Pharmacogenomics in 1959. Pharmacogenomics can be defined as the study of genetic effect on response of a particular drug or drugs. It identifies responders and non-responders to medication. It is relatively new field which combines pharmacology (study of drugs) and genomics (study of gene and their function).

Advantages

- It helps in development of drugs with more therapeutic benefits and reduced damage to the health cells.

- Drugs can be prescribed according to an individual's genetic profile that decreases the possible adverse effects.

- Dosages of the drugs can be determined more accurately.

2.4.4 Proteomics

The term "proteome" was specified by Marc Wilkins in 1994. Proteomics can be defined as the protein complement of the genome, it tells about the two-dimensional gel electrophoresis (2-DE) and quantitative image analysis.2-DE is a method of protein separation; however, it is difficult to identify the proteins through this method.

2.4.5 Array Technology

Array technology depends on the RNA and DNA hybridization reaction. Several genes can be analyzed by array technology. It involves hybridization between two DNA strands. In array technology, sample which contains nucleic acid is labeled and hybridize the sample with the gene specific targets on the array. The array analysis technology provides information on thousands of targets in a single experiment.

2.5   Drug Discovery Cycle

Drug discovery cycle: a general layout of drug discovery cycle is shown in Figure 2.3.

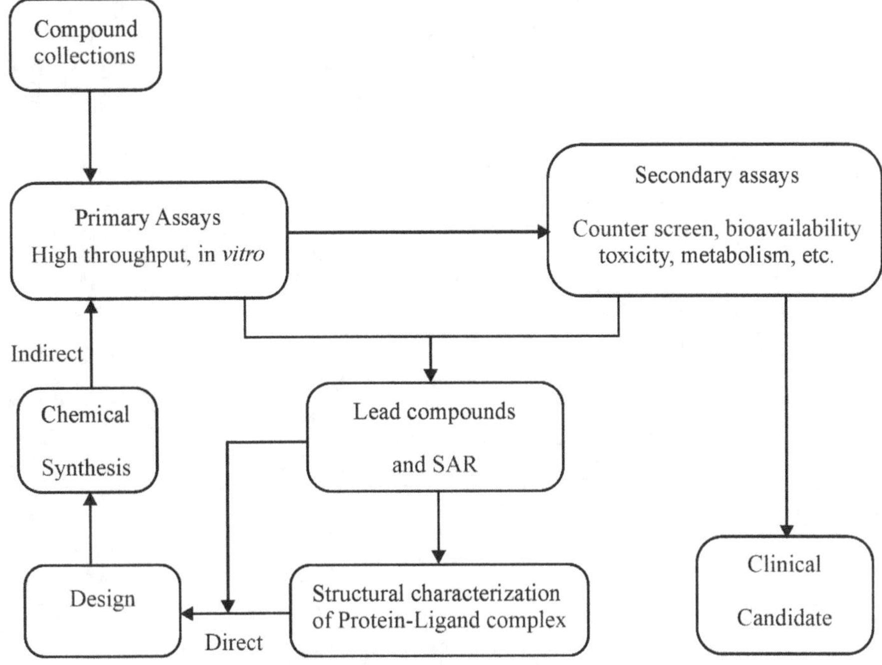

Figure 2.3 Drug discovery cycle.

References

- Grabowski, H., Vernon, J., Di Masi, J. A. Returns on research and development for 1990's new drug introduction. Pharmacoeconomics. 2002; 20 (3):11-29.

- Katzung, B.G., 2007. Basic and clinical pharmacology. In: Masters, S. B., Trevor, A.J., (Eds.), Tata McGraw Hill, Lange Publications. New York ; New Delhi, pp. 69-75.

- Vogel, H.G., 2002. Drug Discovery and evaluation: Pharmacological assays. Springer-Verlag Berlin Heidelberg publication. New York, pp. 1-5.

- Rang, H. P., Dale, M. M., Ritter, J. M., Flower, R. J., Henderson, G., 2015. Rang and Dales Pharmacology. Churchill Livingstone Publication. China, pp. 89-97.

Chapter 3

Bioassay

3.0 Bioassay

Bioassay can be defined as the process of assessment of concentration of unknown compound from any source like physical, chemical or biological system. It can be determined by measuring the magnitude of the test response to that with the response of a standard upon a biological system like microorganisms or cells or animals under predetermined conditions. It can be defined as the scientific experiment for measuring the potency of a substance on a living system. The applications of bioassay involves the determination of purity or biological activity of a substance such as hormone, vitamin, growth factor, etc. Bioassay can be classified into two types viz.

- **Qualitative bioassay** is the assessment of physical effects of unknown compound that may not be quantified e.g. deformity in animals.

- **Quantitative bioassay** is used to quantify the substance for the estimation of concentration or potency by measuring the biological response it produces. e.g. acetylcholine.

3.1 Principles of Bioassay

- It involves the comparison of test with the standard drug to determine the main pharmacological response.

- The dose response curve will run parallel in case where standard and the test samples have same pharmacological effect and hence their potency ratio can be calculated.

- The pharmacological response produced in an experiment should be reproducible under identical conditions e.g. adrenaline increase the blood pressure of animals in a same species under identical conditions of age, weight, strain / breed, sex, etc.

- The selected method should be sensitive, reliable, and reproducible and reduce errors caused by variations in biology and methods.

3.2   Need of Bioassay

- Bioassay helps to determine concentration of the unknown compound in addition to the potency.
- Substances like drugs, vaccines, toxins, disinfectants and antiseptics etc. can be standardized through bioassay.
- Specificity of the compound can also be determined by using bioassay e.g. identification of the type of bacteria for which the suitable drug can be selected.
- Estimation of Vitamin B_{12} can be performed by bioassay.
- Bioassay is reliable option in cases where no physical and chemical assay is available.
- Sometimes the composition of samples are different but biological activities are same e.g. isolation of cardiac glycosides from different sources, catecholamine etc.
- Bioassay is the reliable option where no other methods of assays are available for sample analysis.
- Situations where chemical method is not available or it is too complex to perform or insensitive to low doses.
- Bioassay is suitable for determining side effects and other drug related toxicities.

3.3   Types of Bioassays

Basically there are two types of bioassays as per the technique used in determination of the sample under test.

- End point or quantal assay
- Graded response assay

3.3.1 End Point or Quantal Assay

It is the simplest bioassay, produces 'All or None' response in animals. In this bioassay method either there will be maximum response or there will be no response. In this bioassay the pharmacological effect produced by the threshold dose of the sample is determined and compared with the standard drug or solution. e.g. cardiac arrest produced by digitalis in cats, hypoglycemic convulsions in mice etc.

3.3.2 Graded Response Assay

The response produced in this bioassay is based on the dose of sample as dose of sample increases these is rise in the response. After attaining the particular response there is no increase in response although the dose is increasing, this effect is known as ceiling effect. The curve is obtained by plotting a graph between dose and response on X and Y axis respectively. The curve is sigmoid in shape, however straight line curve is obtained from log (dose).

Concentration of unknown compound

$$= \frac{\text{Threshold dose of standard}}{\text{Threshold dose of test}} \times \text{Concentration of standard}$$

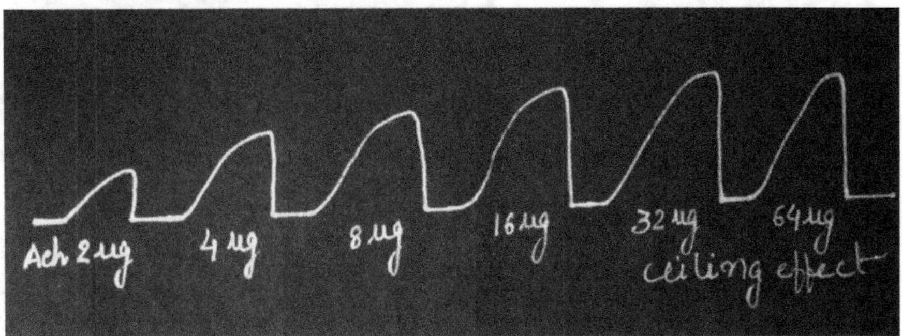

Figure 3.1 Graded response curve.

Graph of graded response assay is depicted in Figure 3.1. The dose of the drug is plotted on X axis and response is plotted on Y axis, get a dose response relationship. Figure 3.1 is a dose response curve (DRC) taken on kymograph paper by rotating drum with the help of writing lever. Graded response assay is of different types.

(a) Matching point or bracketing method

(b) Interpolation bioassay

(c) Three point bioassay

(d) Four point bioassay

(a) **Matching point or bracketing method**: In this method various doses of test is administered and compared with the constant dose of standard in the manner like bracketing by increased and decreased dose of test, this is continued till the standard and test responses are almost identical. Measure the response at equal doses of standard and test and then the effect of standard and test are matched (bracketted) as close as possible. Concentration of unknown sample can be calculated by matching point or bracketing method. Disadvantages of this method are that it is applicable only when the sample of test is too small and it is difficult to estimate margin of error. e.g. posterior pituitary on rat uterus, histamine on guinea pig ileum etc.

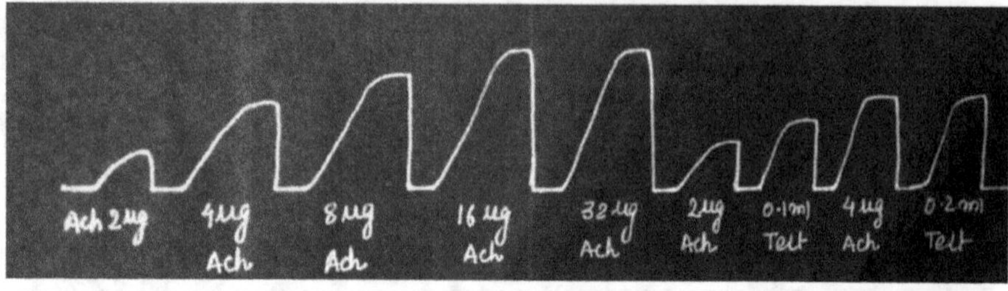

Figure 3.2 Matching point bioassay.

$$\text{Conc. of Unknown} = \frac{\text{Dose of Standard (volume)}}{\text{Dose of Test (volume)}} \times \text{Conc. of Standard}$$

Matching point bioassay is shown in Figure 3.2.

(b) Interpolation bioassay: In this bioassay the quantity of preparation of unknown potency which produces significant effect on test animals or isolated organs or tissues under standard conditions is determined. The response produced by the unknown is expressed as a percentage response as that of standard and the amount of test compound required to produce the same pharmacological response as standard is compared. Graph of interpolation assay is shown in Figure 3.3. In this method dose response curve (DRC) of standard is obtained as discussed under "graded response assay" till the ceiling effect is obtained. Then, one or two responses due to unknown drug is recorded. The graph of log (dose) vs percent response of standard is plotted (standard curve) and the corresponding concentration of unknown is obtained from standard curve by interpolation.

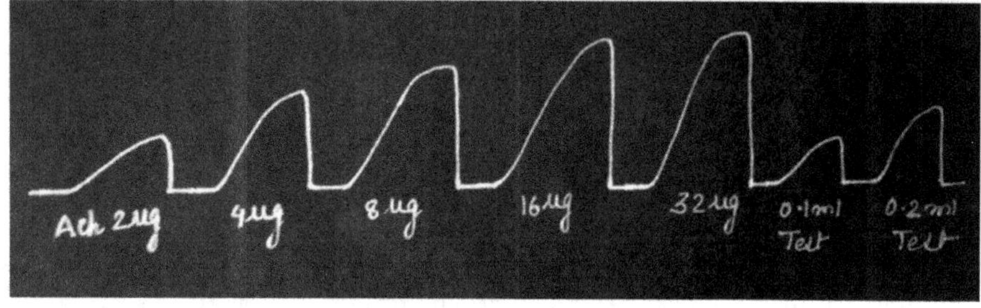

Figure 3.3 Interpolation bioassay.

3.3.3 Multi Point Bioassay

This bioassay involves both interpolation and bracketing method. It can be further divided into different point bioassays such as 3 point (2+1), 4 point (2+2) and 6 point (3+3) bioassay.

(c) **Three point bioassay (2+1 dose assay)** - It is fast & convenient method indicates two response of Standard (S) and one response of Test (T). Three point bioassay is depicted in Figure 3.4.

- **Methodology:** First the DRC of standard is obtained as discussed under "graded response assay" till the ceiling effect is obtained. Log dose response (LDR) curve is plotted with different concentration of standard drug solutions and given test solution. Two doses in ml of standard as s_1 and s_2 is selected in the ratio of 2:3 from linear part of LDR and get the responses S_1 and S_2 (height, mm) respectively. One test dose in ml (t) and s (ml) selected and get the response T (height, mm) between S_1 and S_2. Response is recorded in three sets by using Latin square design in any combination such as.

  - S_1 S_2 T
  - T S_1 S_2
  - S_2 S_1 T

Where, S1 and S2: Response in "mm" due to standard dose 1 and 2, lower and higher value respectively.

T: Response due to test dose in "mm"

s1 and s2 : Dose in "ml" of standard dose 1 and 2.

t: dose in "ml" of test

$$\text{Calculation: Log Potency ratio}[M] = \frac{(T-S1)}{(S2-S1)} \times \log \frac{s2}{s1}$$

$$\text{Concentration of unknown} = \frac{s1}{t} \text{anti} \log[M]$$

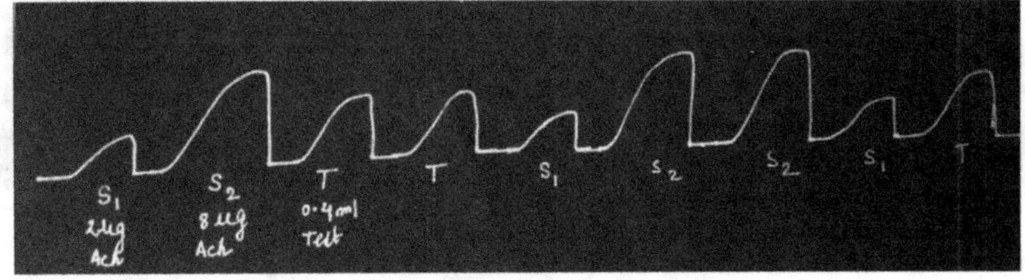

Figure 3.4 Three point bioassay.

(d) **Four point bioassay [2 +2 dose assay]:** It indicates two response of Standard (S) and two response of Test (T) (e.g., Ach bioassay). Four point bioassay is depicted in Figure 3.5.

- **Methodology:** First the DRC of standard is obtained as discussed under "graded response assay" till the ceiling effect is achieved.

The log dose response curve is plotted between different concentration of standard solutions and the given test solution. Two doses in "ml" of standard i.e. s_1 and s_2 are selected from linear part of DRC and the response in "mm", height S1 and S2 is recorded. Two test doses in "ml" t_1 and t_2 are selected and get response in "mm", height T1 and T2 between S1 and S2. Data is recorded in four sets in any combination by using Latin square method such as:

- S1 T2 T1 S2

- S2 S1 T2 T1

- T1 S2 S1 T2

- S1 S2 T1 T2

Where, S1 and S2: Response in "mm" due to standard dose 1 and 2, i.e lower and higher dose respectively.

T1 and T2: Response in "mm" due to test dose 1 and 2. i.e lower and higher dose respectively.

s1 and s2: Dose in "ml" of standard 1 and 2. i.e lower and higher dose respectively.

t1 and t2: Dose in "ml" of test 1 and 2. i.e lower and higher dose respectively.

$$\text{Calculation: Log Potency ratio}[M] = \frac{(T_1 - S1) - (T2 - S2)}{(S_2 - S1) - (T2 - T1)} \times \log \frac{s2}{s1}$$

$$\text{Concentration of unknown} = \frac{s1}{t1} \text{anti} \log[M]$$

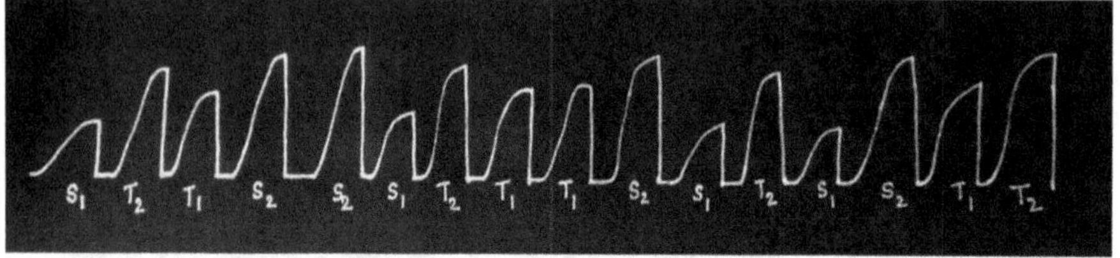

Figure 3.5 Four Point Bioassay.

3.4   Basic Procedure of Recording DRC (Student Organ Bath)

Student organ bath is set up with outer jacket filled with water and temperature of water is maintained at 37°C. Student organ bath is shown in Figure 3.6 and Sherrington drum (kymograph) is depicted in Figure 3.7. Organ tube is filled with physiological salt solution (PSS) according to the tissue preparation and it is attached with a reservoir which is also filled with PSS. PSS is passed in to organ tube in which tissue is mounted. Tissue should be of optimum size of about 1.0 to 1.5cm. The thread is passed through the lumen of the tissue. While passing the thread care must be taken that lumen of the tissue should not be closed. Tissue tying technique is depicted in Figure 3.8. One end of the lumen is tied to the oxygen tube and another end to the writing lever (here frontal writing level). Counter balance the tissue weight by using the clay. Tissue is allowed to relax for 30 minute and PSS is changed in every 5 min interval. Kymograph paper is pasted on Sherrington's drum. Drum is set at speed of 0.25 mm/sec. After the tissue gets relaxed, the base line is plotted for 30 sec by switching on the kymograph. Rotating drum and lever should be aligned in the same plane. First dose of drug is injected and response is recorded with contact time of 90 sec. During recording of response weight is lifted up (after load, stretching tension). Consecutive washing is given to the tissue so as to negate the effect of previous drug. Again a baseline of 30 sec is recorded. Second dose of the same drug or another drug is injected and response is recoded of 90 sec. Again the tissue is washed and following procedure is repeated until the ceiling effect or desired effect is achieved. At the end the kymograph paper is removed and tracings is fixed with the help of shellac solution (fixing solution).

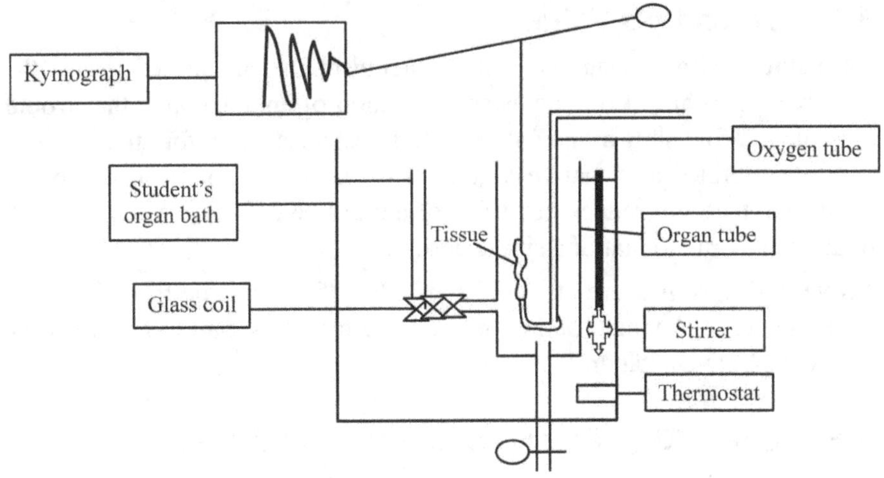

Figure 3.6 Student organ bath.

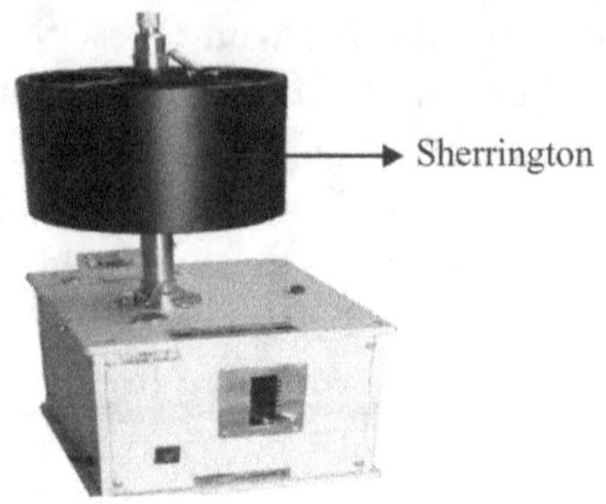

Figure 3.7 Kymograph.

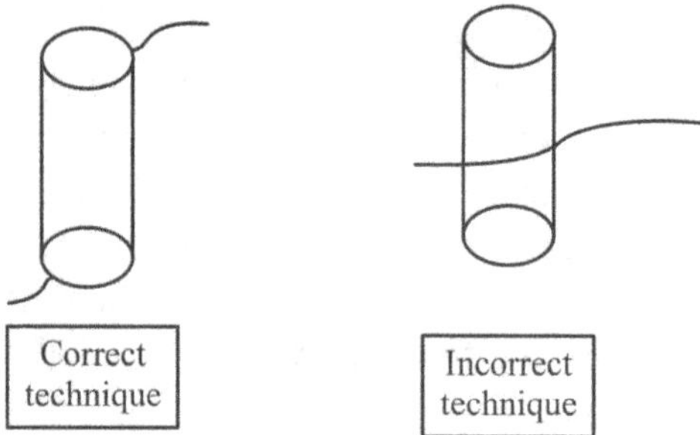

Figure 3.8 Technique to tie tissue.

3.5 pA and pD Value

pA value-It is a measure of drug antagonism. It can be defined as the negative logarithm of the molar concentration of an antagonist that would produce a 2-fold shift in the concentration response curve for an agonist or It is also defined as negative logarithm of the molar concentration of an antagonist that will reduce the effect of a multiple dose x (usually 2 or 10) of an active drug to that of a single dose.

pD value-It is a measure of agonist affinity. It is calculated from the dose-response curve. Agonists acting on the same receptors may have same pA_x with competitive antagonist.

3.6 LD$_{50}$, ED$_{50}$, Therapeutic Index and IC$_{50}$

LD$_{50}$ – It is the amount of test substance which causes death of 50% of subjects taking it. In LD_{50}, LD refers to lethal dose. Acute toxicity or short term poisoning is measured by LD_{50}. Oral and dermal route for administration of test compound is found to be most common route for determination of LD_{50} (Figure 3.9). The test was created by J.W. Trevan in 1927.

ED$_{50}$ – It is the effective dose of drug that produces therapeutic response in 50% of the subjects involved in the study.

Therapeutic index: It is measure of safety of a drug. It is the ratio of LD$_{50}$ to ED$_{50}$.

$$\text{Therapeutic index (TI)} = \frac{LD_{50}}{ED_{50}}$$

The greater the index, safer is the compound.

IC$_{50}$-It is half of the maximum inhibitory concentration. It is defined as the measure of potency of a substance that inhibits the half of the specific population or biological function of any organism.

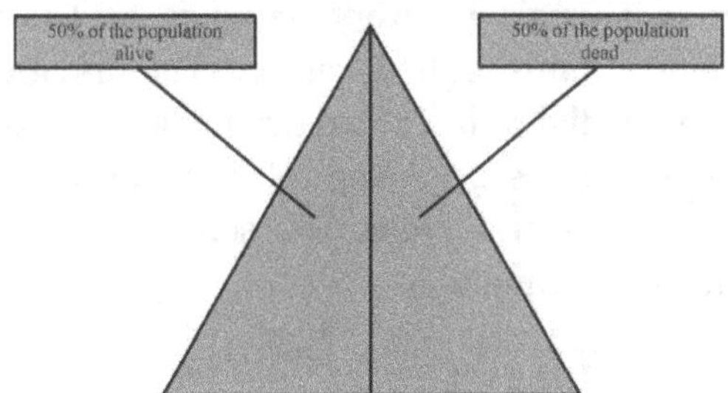

Figure 3.9 LD$_{50}$ determination.

3.6.1 Importance of LD$_{50}$

It was very complex to compare toxicities caused by different chemicals. LD$_{50}$ tests are now employed to measure the quantity of the chemical that may cause death. It has importance in comparing the intensity and toxic potency of several chemicals.

3.6.2 Uses of LD$_{50}$

- To establish industrial exposure limits.
- To develop transportation regulations.
- To establish safety guidelines for the appropriate use of clothing and equipment.
- To establish emergency procedures in case of accident.

Note: Toxicity of any chemical depends on the value of LD$_{50}$, its higher value indicates the chemical is less toxic however its lower value indicates the chemical is much toxic. Acute toxicity can be determined through LD$_{50}$ on animals of particular strain, sex and age. Two most common method of detection are:

- ➤ Hodge and Sterner Scale
- ➤ Gosselin, Smith and Hodge Scale

3.6.3 Methods to Determine LD_{50}

Different methods are used to determine LD_{50} are as follow:

(a) Arithmetical method of Karber

(b) Graphical method of Miller and Tainter method

(c) Lorkes's method

(d) Up and down procedure

(e) Fixed dose method (FDP)

(f) Reed-Muench method

(a) Arithmetic method of Karber

The number of animals in every group is 5. The response should satisfy the Gaussian distribution roughly. The first group of animals is administered with the vehicle and from the second group different doses of test substances are given to the animals. The dose must be increased with geometric proportion series. LD_{50} is determined by using the following formula.

$$LD_{50} = LD_{100} - \left[\frac{a \times b}{n} \right]$$

Where LD_{50} = lethal dose 50 or median lethal dose

LD_{100} = the dose required to kill 100% of the population or microorganisms.

a = difference in dose

b = mean mortality value

n = group population

- **Disadvantage**: Too many animals are sacrificed in this method.

(b) Graphical method of Miller and Tainter method

Percentage mortality is determined by its conversion into probit. Observed values are plotted against log (dose). LD_{50} and its simultaneous standard error are determined through the graph, if the line is straight enough.

- **Disadvantage:** Too many animals are sacrificed in this method.

(c) Lorkes's Method

This method is divided into two phases, Phase 1- nine animals are selected and divided into 3 groups each containing three animals. Different doses of test substances are given to the animals i.e. 10,100 and 1000 mg/kg of test substance. Animals are observed for 24 hours to monitor general behavior and any mortality.

Phase 2: It requires 3 groups of animals. Each group contains one animal. High doses (1600, 2900 and 5000 mg/kg) of the test substances are given to the animals. Animals are observed for 24 hours to monitor general behavior and any mortality.

$$LD_{50} = \sqrt{(D_0 \times D_{100})}$$

Where D_0 = highest dose that gave no mortality

D_{100} = lowest dose that produced mortality

- **Advantage:** Fewer animals are sacrificed.
- **Disadvantages:** Reproducibility, reliability and accuracy are questionable.

A comparison between all these methods is shown in Table 3.1

Table 3.1 Comparison of the methods

Particulars	Method of Karber	Method of Miller and Tainter	Method of Lorke
Number of animals used	More than required	More than required	Appropriate
Expenditure	High	High	Average
Accuracy of results	Inaccurate	Inaccurate	Doubtful

(d) Up and down procedure

It is used to assess acute toxicity. In this procedure animals are administered a drug one at a time. If at that particular dose animals survive then the dose is increased. If the increased dose causes the death of the animal, dose is decreased.

(e) Fixed dose method (FDP)

Fixed dose procedure (FDP) is used to assess acute oral toxicity of all kind of substance. In this method test substance is administered in the dose of 5, 50,500 and 2000 mg/kg. Test substance is administered to 5 males and 5 females. The main aim is to evaluate a dose which produces clear sign of toxicity but at this dose there is no mortality. On the basis of the result of the first test, further testing at higher or lower dose is necessary. If mortality occurs at initial lower dose, then further testing at higher dose is compulsory.

(f) Reed-Muench method

It is used to evaluate 50% end point in experimental biology. This method assess about LD_{50}, EC_{50} (half maximal effective) and IC_{50} (inhibitory concentration).

References

- Arunlakshana, O., Schild, H. O. Some quantitative uses of drug antagonists.Br J Pharmacol.1959; 14 (1): 48-58.

- Kulkarni, S. K., 1999. Hand Book of Experimental Pharmacology. Vallabh Prakashan. Delhi. pp. 11-15.

- Chinedu, E., Arome, D., Ameh, S. F. New Method for determining acute toxicity in animal models. Toxicol Int. 2013; 20 (3): 224-226.

- Bodakhe, S.H., Gupta S.K. 2016 A Text Book of Experimental Pharmacology. Dhawan publications. Delhi. pp.133-135.

- Muthannan, A.R., Determination of 50% endpoint titer using a simple formula. World J Virol. 2016; 5(2): 85–86.

- Bruce, R.D. An up-and-down procedure for acute toxicity testing. FundamAppl Toxicol.1985; 5(1):151-7.

Chapter 4

Evaluation of Drugs acting on Autonomic Nervous System

4.0 Experimental Models of Drugs Acting on the Parasympathetic Nervous System

4.1 Parasympathomimetic System

Compounds which have an affinity for cholinergic receptors are known as parasympathomimetic agents or cholinomimetic agents. They mimic the actions of acetylcholine. There are three kinds of parasympathomimetic agents:

- Indirectly acting agents which increase the concentration of acetylcholine

- Directly acting agents which directly bind with the receptor

- Those reacting with other receptors, i.e., receptors in the system which is not affected by acetylcholine (barium chloride).

4.1.1 Isolated Eye of Rodents

Background: This model is useful to screen parasympathomimetic drugs and is a widely accepted model.

Methodology

Rats, mice or guinea pigs with pigmented iris are selected. Animals are sacrificed, and their eyeballs are removed and enucleated with the help of blunt, curved surgical scissors. The eyes are kept in Krebs-Ringer solution and then mounted in appropriately sized, hemispherical sockets, set in black lucite trays. Trays are dipped in bicarbonate buffered Krebs ringer solution. This is fixed on the stage of the microscope. This mixture is bubbled with 95% oxygen and 5% carbon dioxide. The pH is maintained at 7.4. Pupillary diameter is observed with a microscope. The eyes are placed in the chamber, and after a 30 min period for stabilization of the preparation, the pupillary diameter is measured as a control. Krebs solution is replaced with fresh Krebs solution, and it contains the predetermined concentration of the test solution. The pupillary diameter is then measured after 30 min. The response is expressed as a ratio of this diameter to the control diameter.

Evaluation: The plot of this ratio against the logarithm of the molar concentration of the test substance is a straight line.

4.2   Parasympatholytics

Parasympatholytic agents are also known as anticholinergic or antimuscarinic agents. They antagonize the actions of acetylcholine. Their activity may be evidenced by mydriasis and by inhibition of the secretions of the digestive tract (saliva, gastric juice, etc.).

Experimental models

- Mydriasis
- Rectus muscle of the frog

4.2.1 Mydriasis

Background: A qualitative test for mydriasis may be part of the procedure for blind screening. Mice are most often used for studying mydriasis activity, but rabbits are also used.

Requirements: Mice (15-16 g, either sex) dissecting microscope, glass jars.

Methodology:

Experimental arrangement: The mice are placed singly in glass jars on a white table, beneath a fluorescent light in an otherwise dark room.

Observation: After half an hour the pupil diameter of the mice is measured by means of a graduated scale with the eyepiece of a dissecting microscope.

Administration of drug: Test drug is given through i.p. route at a dose of 0.01 ml/g of body weight.

Pupil diameter: Pupil diameter is again determined after 10, 20 and 30 min. A group of 5 mice is used for each dose level.

Evaluation: Drugs that block the parasympathetic ganglia cause dilatation of the pupil in mammals, where the circular fibers of the iris are unstriated muscles.

4.2.2 Rectus Muscle of the Frog

Background: Local anesthetics, analgesics, and substances having quinidine-like activity may owe their properties to their antagonism of acetylcholine.

Requirements: Frog, ringer solution, acetylcholine, organ bath

Methodology:

Selection of animals: Frog of an appropriate weight

Suspension of tissue: Suspension of tissues is prepared placing the isolated frog rectus muscle in a bath containing frog ringer solution (7 ml).

Replacement of fluid: The fluid is replaced every 5 min by frog Ringer solution containing acetylcholine.

Recording: The stimulant effect of this ester is recorded for 90 sec with the aid of a lever and kymograph.

Measurement: This response to acetylcholine is constant, but is observed three times at the beginning of each experiment.

Administration of drug: The drug is administered to animals after 90 sec prior to the addition of acetylcholine. The fluid containing test solution is also changed.

Evaluation: The concentration of a test substance required to decrease the effect of acetylcholine is recorded, or the concentration to diminish the response by 50% is recorded.

4.3   Sympathomimetics

Adrenaline is the primary neurotransmitter of the adrenergic system. It produces various interventions such as mydriasis in eye, stimulation of the heart, dilatation of the coronary arteries, rise in blood pressure, constriction of capillaries in the skin and mucosa, relaxation of bronchial muscles, contraction of gastrointestinal sphincters, constriction of pulmonary vessels and splenic capsule, inhibition of gastric secretion, stimulation of the uterus, glycogenolysis in the liver etc.

4.3.1 Uterus and Ascending Colon of the Rat

Background: The rat uterus is sensitive to adrenaline. It can show spontaneous activity.

Requirement: Female Albino rats (160-170 g), acetylcholine, adrenaline

Methodology:

Apparatus: Temperature of the bath is maintained at 29-30°C. Larger uteri are more sensitive than smaller. Uterus is mounted in the organ bath.

Induction of contraction: Acetylcholine (0.5 to 1.0 µg) is added to the bath every 2 min and washed out when the effect is maximal (30 to 40 sec). Adrenaline(0.21 ml)is administered to the bath 1 min before a dose of acetylcholine. Another dose of adrenaline is given as soon as the effect of acetylcholine becomes normal.

Note:

- Screening the lowest dose of adrenaline or test substance causing the response to acetylcholine to be reduced by one-half is taken as a measure of the adrenaline-like activity.

- Noradrenaline is comparatively inactive on this preparation.

4.4   Sympatholytics

Substances that inhibit the mediation of neurotransmitter in the brain are called adrenergic-blocking agents, adrenaline antagonists, adrenolytic agents, and sympatholytic agents.

Experimental model

- Blood pressure of the rat
- α- Sympatholytic activity in isolated vascular smooth muscle
- β_1- Sympatholytic activity in isolated guinea pig atria

4.4.1 Blood Pressure of the Rat

Requirements: Albino rats (180-240 g), anesthetic agents.

Anesthesia: Urethane or any other suitable anesthetic agent is used.

Measurement of blood pressure: Blood pressure (BP) is measured with a mercury manometer connected to a cannula in the carotid artery or by noninvasive techniques like noninvasive blood pressure (NIBP) apparatus.

Evaluation: The effective dose of any drug is expressed as the activity dose coefficient or ADC, which is the product of the maximal depression of the blood pressure in millimeters and the time interval of depression in minutes, divided by twice the dose in mg or kg.

4.4.2 α- Sympatholytic Activity in Isolated Vascular Smooth Muscle

Background: Antiadrenergic drugs such as phentolamine decreases vascular tone by blocking the α-adrenergic receptor. In this experimental model the adrenergic agonist drugs can be screened that reduces vascular smooth muscle contractions.

Requirements: Guinea pigs (400 g, any sex) or Sprague Dawley rats (180-250 g), Krebs-Henseleit buffer solution, 11.5 M glucose, noradrenalineHCl,

Methodology: Exsanguinations and stunning techniques are used to sacrifice animals followed by isolation of thoracic aorta or pulmonary artery and cut into helical strips (1-2 mm width and 15-20 mm length). These strips are mounted in an organ bath containing Krebs-Henseleit buffer solution made up of 11.5 M glucose (37°C). Noradrenaline is administered repeatedly to induce contraction to pulmonary artery or the thoracic aorta.

The cumulative doses of test and standard (phentolamine) drugs are loaded into the organ bath after achieving a stable plateau of identical sized contractions. The test drugs are given in consecutive concentrations when the response of the previous dose has reached a plateau. However, pre- and post-drug administration the contractile force is determined. The percentage inhibition is calculated as produced by test drug in the form of spasmogen-induced contractions and compare it with the maximal contraction with a spasmogen alone.

4.4.3 β1- Sympatholytic Activity in Isolated Guinea Pig Atria

Background:

The β-agonist drugs increases the force of contraction of right atria and stimulates isolated left atria by potentiating contractions. β-sympatholytic activity acts as antagonists and blocks the action produced by β-agonist drugs. These effects can be evaluated in isolated right and left guinea pig atria. β1-antagonistic activity can be assessed by this test because predominant β1-adrenoreceptors are found in heart.

Requirements: Guinea pigs (250–300 g, either sex), Krebs-Henseleit buffer solution, 11.5 M glucose.

Methodology

Exsanguinations and stunning techniques are used to sacrifice animals followed by isolation of right or the left atrium and then mounted in a 50 ml organ bath with a preload of 100 mg.

Mounting of tissue: The strips are mounted in an organ bath containing Krebs-Henseleit buffer solution made up of 11.5 M glucose (37°C) and aerated with 95% O_2 and 5% CO_2.

Induction of contraction:

- **Right atrium**

  Isoprenaline is administered into the organ bath after 30 min of equilibration period to potentiate inotropic action and frequency of the isolated right atrium. Repeated doses of isoprenaline are added with the starting dose of 0.05 µg/ml consecutively at 3 min of intervals.

- **Left atrium**

  Square wave stimulator is used to stimulate left atrium; the condition of stimulation is wave of 2 impulses/s at a voltage of 15 V for duration of 1 ms after an equilibration period of 30 min. β-agonist isoprenaline is added at concentrations of 0.05–0.1 mg/ml.

Administration of the drug: The organ bath is thoroughly flushed for 1 min after getting a plateau of isoprenaline administration followed by addition of test compound. Isoprenaline is added again after 5 min. The standard drugs used for β_1-Sympatholytic activity are propranolol HCl, amrinone, milrinone, etc.

Efficacy of test drug: β-receptor blocking activity of the test compound produces following effects:

- Same potentiation of inotropy and frequency is produced by higher isoprenaline concentrations.

- The increase in inotropy and frequency is reduced with the same isoprenaline concentrations added as before.

Evaluation: Percentage inhibition of increased inotropy and frequency by test drug due to electrical stimulation or isoprenaline is calculated and compared to pre-drug activity. Change in percent = refractory period is calculated.

References

- Zangeneh, F. Z., Naghizadeh, M. M. Locus coeruleus lesions, and PCOS: the role of the central and peripheral sympathetic nervous system in the ovarian function of the rat.IJRM. 2012; 10(2): 113–120.

- Zygmunt, A., Stanczyk, J. Methods of evaluation of autonomic nervous system function, Arch Med Sci. 2010; 6, 1: 11-18.

- Gupta, S. K., 2004. Drug screening methods. Jaypee brothers medical publishers LTD. New Delhi. pp. 37-44.

Chapter 5

Evaluation of Drugs Acting on Central Nervous System

5.1 Anti-Anxiety Activity

Anxiety is the condition of behavioral inhibition due to changing circumstances or environmental events that are punishing, non-rewarding or novel. Anti-anxiety screening models are used to screen novel or lead compounds for determination of anxiogenic or anxiolytic activities. These models can be divided into the following broad categories:

5.1.1 Experimental Models

(a) Social interaction induced anxiety

Background: In this experimental model the pair of rats are allowed to spend time on social interaction that decreases the anxiety of rats. The experimental conditions can be changed by changing the intensity of light and familiarization of the test arena. However, bright light and unfamiliarity of the test arena may be used to induce anxiety. On the basis of these conditions, four test conditions are defined i.e. low light, unfamiliar arena; low light, familiar arena; high light, unfamiliar arena and high light, familiar arena. It has seen that the scoring of control animals are highest in low light and familiar test arena in comparison to low light, unfamiliar condition or high light, familiar test conditions. The anti anxiety drug (Benzodiazepine) increases the social interaction in rats in low light and familiar condition.

Requirements: Male or female Albino rats weighing (150-170 g), testing drugs, saline, animal cages, test arena with video camera that is away from disturbances, the specification of test arena should have wooden box (60 × 60 cm) with 35 cm high walls and infrared photocells mounted in the walls (4.5 and 12.5 cm) from the floor, the illumination in the test arena may be either bright (300 radiometric lux) or dim (30 radiometric lux) [Figure 5.1 (a) and (b)].

Methodology

Acclimatization: Animals are allowed to stay individually in separate cages 5 days before the experiment and each rat weighed daily. Food and water provided *ad libitum* with low light (50 lux).

Test arena: The test arena is placed in the quiet room that is equipped with video camera mounted vertically above the test arena.

Treatment: House rats in adjacent cages and allocate them to test conditions and /or drug treatments. Place the animals in the test arena individually for familiarization with the arena for 10 min on 2 consecutive days. The test arena then move to the dim light for 60 min before administration of test drugs.

Administration of drug: Test and standard drugs are given intravenously in the dim light area.

Test conditions: Any one test conditions depending upon light frequency and familiarity with test arena can be selected as selected above depending upon the purpose of the experiment.

Recording: The recording is done by the camera placed above the test arena and it can be observed on a screen in an adjacent room.

Scoring: Scoring is performed according to the time spent in active social interaction. It helps to identify aggressive and non-aggressive behavior of animals. Aggressive behavior may be wrestling, boxing, kicking, etc. and non-aggressive behavior may be grooming, sniffing, etc.

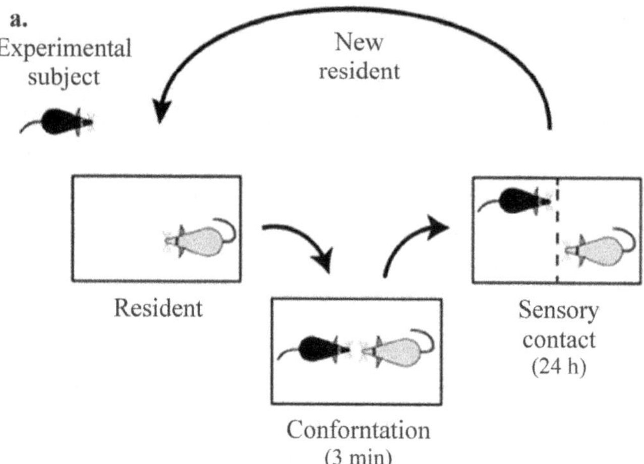

b.

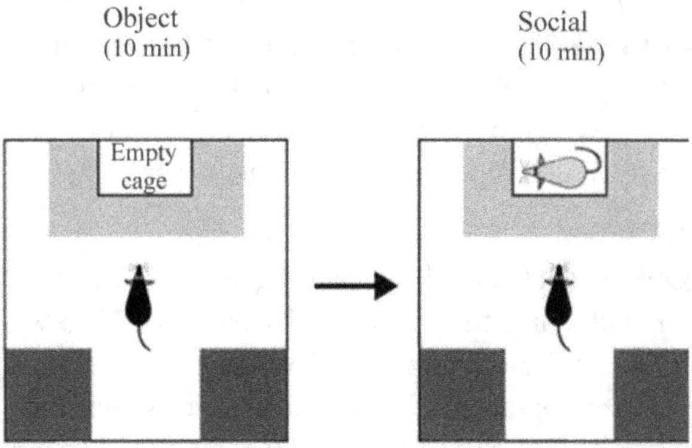

Object
(10 min)

Social
(10 min)

Empty cage

Figure 5.1 (a) Infrared photocell mounted with illumination.
(b) Wooden box for interaction.

(b) Yohimbine induced convulsions

Background: Potential anxiolytic and GABA-mimetic drugs shows antagonism of Yohimbine-induced seizures in mice.

Requirements: Swiss male mice (20-30 g), yohimbine hydrochloride

Methodology

Administration of drug: Animals are placed individually in transparent propylene cages, and test and reference drugs are administered intraperitonealy, 30 min prior to the induction of anxiety.

Induction of anxiety: Anxiety is induced by injection through subcutaneous route, Yohimbine hydrochloride at a dose of 45 mg/kg.

Observation: The animals are observed for onset of any seizure or number of clonic seizures for 60 min.

(c) Foot shock induced aggression

Background: Animals are given electric shock, and they show aggression and defensive behavior [Fig. 5.2].

Requirements: Swiss albino mice or Wistar albino rats

Methodology
Procedure: The electric shock is supplied to the hind paws of experimental animals by placing them in a box containing grid floor with steel rods at a distance of 6 mm. These steel rods induces foot shock or aggression due to induction of pain by supplying a constant current of 0.6 or 0.8 mA. The protocol follows current delivery of 60-Hz current for 5s, then pause current for 5s and continue upto 3 min.

Same responses can be obtained by giving certain drugs like apomorphine and mescaline to the pairs of animals.

Observations: The attacking behavior of animals to each other is observed. The fight between animals is recorded for 3 min. The fighting behavior may be considered to leaping, vocalizing, rearing, running or attacking to another animals by boxing, biting, or hitting.

Advantage

ED_{50} can be determined by handing the forelimbs of animals from a thin bar and bring their hind limbs on to the bar within a stipulated time frame. It is determined to lower the number of fights by 50% or to determine paralysis in animals. The specificity of antidefense effects can be calculated by dividing the ED_{50} of number of fights to the ED_{50} for paralysis. Good antidefense specificity is based on high ratio; however, lower values indicates strong interfering effects. Neuroleptics show this ratio less than one, tricyclic antidepressants show ratio more than 1, however, benzodiazepines also show ratio less than 1 because of their muscle relaxation property.

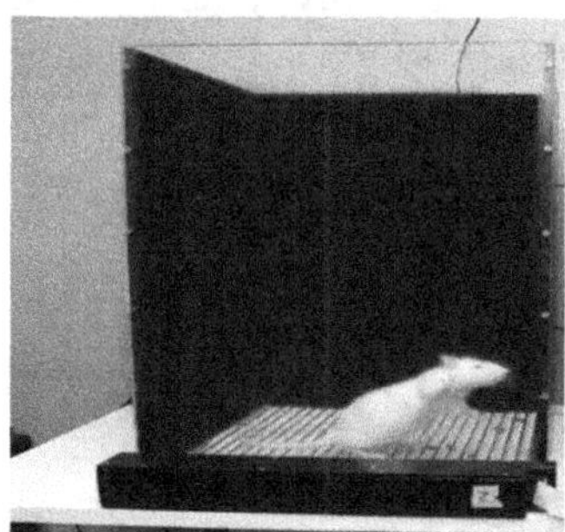

Figure 5.2 Foot shock induced aggression.

(d) Light and dark exploratory model

Background: This experimental model helps to define conflict tendencies between mice. It is a simple behavioral model helps in screen of anxiolytic drugs according to Crawley and Goodwin (1980). In this model, animals are allowed to move between bright and dark fields. The crossing of animals and locomotor activity is enhanced between these two chambers after anxiolytic drugs administration. The number of crossings is noted between the two chambers. It is correlated with other behavior of the animals that is not related to the locomotor activity in bright field or open field [Figure 5.3].

Requirements: Dark room, test drugs, animals, saline

Test apparatus: A polypropylene animal cage with dimensions of 44 × 21 × 21 cm. The cage is darkened with black spray over one-third of its surface and a partition is made with 13 cm long × 5 cm high opening. This partition is used for separating the dark part from bright part.

Methodology

Selection of animals: Naive mice or rats 6-8 animals in each group.

Administration of drug: The test drug is given through intra-peritoneal route before 30 min of commencement of the experiment.

Observation: Then animals are placed in the cage and observed for 10 min.

Calculation: The dose response curve is plotted at last for determination of number of crossings in comparison to the total activity counts during the 10 min.

Note: The apparatus should be washed after each trial, any faeces, urine or dirt should be cleaned.

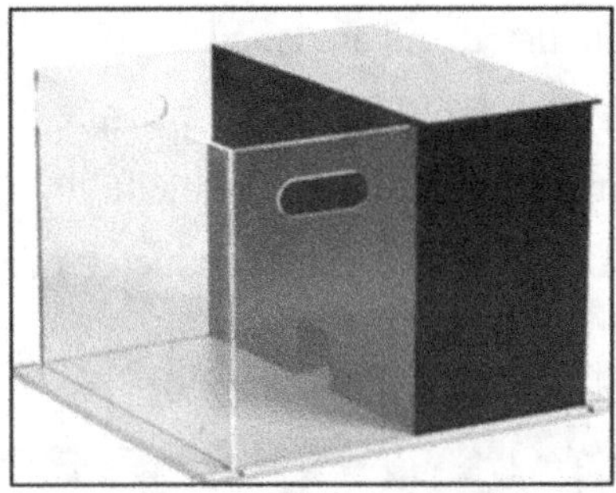

Figure 5.3 Light and dark model.

(e) Elevated plus maze test

Background: This method was introduced by Mantgomery (1958) for evaluation of anxiolytic and anxiogenic drugs. Anxiolytic drugs increase the open arm exploration time by decreasing anxiety whereas the anxiogenic drugs have on the contrary an opposite effect [Figure 5.4].

Requirements: Wistar rats (200-250 g), test room without any noise and away from disturbance equipped with video camera for recording.

Apparatus: The elevated plus-maze consists of two open and two enclosed arms each of 50 × 10 × 40 cm dimensions with an open roof arranged in such a manner that the two open arms should be opposite to each other.

Methodology

Acclimatization: Animals are acclimatized to the laboratory conditions 10 days prior to the experiment. They should be handled by the researchers in alternate days to acclimatize them and making favorable with the laboratory conditions.

The setting of Apparatus: The plus maze apparatus should be placed at the height of 40-60 cm from the floor and mount the camera above the maze.

Administration of drugs: The test drug and standard are administered to the animals by intraperitoneal route before 30 min to experiment.

Observation: Animals placed in the center of the maze and observe them for the next 5 min and measure the following:

- Number of entries into open arms and closed arms separately
- Time spent in open arms, closed arms and central square separately

Calculation: the ratio of open or closed arm time to the total arm entries/time is calculated and analyzed.

Advantage: It is considered a reliable measure of antianxiety activity.

Disadvantage: It is a time consuming method.

Caution: The procedure should be conducted in a sound-proof room.

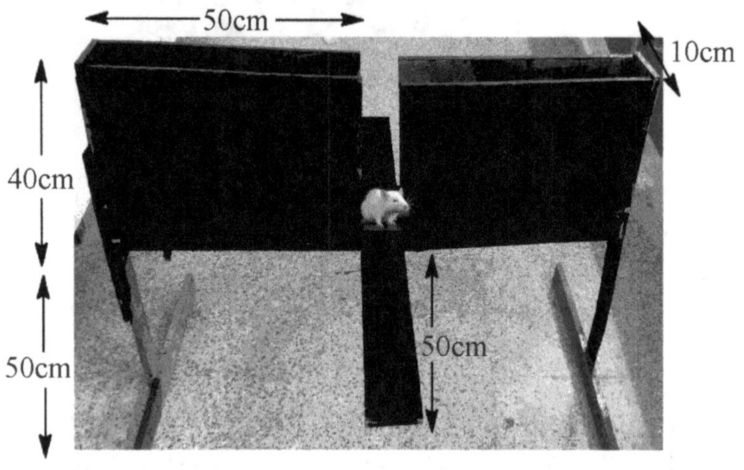

Figure 5.4 Elevated plus-maze apparatus.

(f) Isolation induced aggression behavior

Background: Aggression is developed due to long term isolation from other animals. Thus, compounds are screened for anti-aggression activity using this model.

Procedure: Animals are kept in isolated cages for 6 weeks before experiment and their aggressive behavior is tested before administration of drug. Two animals of same sex are kept in one cage to accustom for 5 minute.

Observations: The aggression of isolated animal is observed as hitting the tail, biting and screaming to other animal. It can be evaluated for test drug after 30, 60 and 120 min of subcutaneous route and 60, 120 and 240 min of oral route. The behavior of animals is changed after treatment with CNS acting drugs.

Evaluation: Complete suppression of fighting behavior between the animals is calculated and reduced aggressiveness reaction time in animals is noted.

(g) Defensive Burying

Background: This experimental model do not require initial training of animals. Electric shock is provided through electrified probe, it is attached to the wall of the test chamber. Animals reflexively withdraw from the probe and then approach to the probe slowly; snout first in a low voice followed by elongated posture by abrupt withdrawals. The animals start to spray bedding material rapidly with alternating thrusts from the floor to the chamber and over the probe using forepaws. Defensive burying is suppressed by antianxiety drugs in a dose-dependent manner that is accompained with enhanced number of probe shocks.

Requirements: Swiss albino mice (20-30 g) or Wistar rats (180-250 g), drugs to be tested, saline, bedding material, aspen chips, quiet room, video camera, and shock-probe test apparatus.

Methodology

Acclimatization: Animals housed individually in cages and maintained on 12 h light/dark cycle with adequate supply of food and water.

Habituation: Habituate individuals or groups of animals by placing them in the test chamber, 30 min prior to the commencement of experiment on each of 4 consecutive days.

Administration of drug: Administer drugs intravenously before performing test, insert the shock probe 6 cm into the plexiglass chamber and secure in place.

Shock treatment: Rats are placed in test chamber that is away from the shock probe. The probe is activated when animal snout or approaching towards probe. Shock intensity 1-2 mA, until rat's reflexive withdrawal from the probe.

Recording: The recording parameters are as follows:

- Duration of burying (time of spraying bedding by animals towards probe)
- Number of contact-induced shocks
- Scoring of behavioral reaction to shock on four points:

    1 = flinch of head or forepaw

    2 = whole body flinch away from the probe

    3 = whole body flinch followed by walking towards probe

    4 = whole body flinch followed by quick running in the opposite side of the chamber's end

- Complete absence of body movement as duration of immobility
- The treatment is terminated after 15 min and probe is switched off.

5.2   Antidepressant Activity

Depression is the condition associated with loss of interest, gloomy mood, failure of energy, feeling of guilt, worthlessness, retardation of motor activity, agitation, etc. Emotional symptoms include misery, apathy and pessimism, low self-esteem, indecisiveness and loss of motivation. Biological symptoms include disturbance of sleep, loss of sexual desire, loss of hunger and retardation of thought and action.

Antidepressants are the drugs used for mood elevation, these include monoamine oxidase (MAO) inhibitors, 5-HT and noradrenaline reuptake inhibitors. Various antidepressant drugs like imipramine, amitriptyline, amoxapine, citalopram, reboxetine are used to relieve depression.

Stress is the leading cause for generation of depression which leads to secretion of cortisol followed by cortisol releasing factor (CRF) and adrenocorticotrophic hormone (ACTH). The release of cortisol causes neural apoptosis, in addition to this stress induces excitation of NMDA receptors, it results into apoptosis in brain regions. Pathophysiology of depression is shown in Figure 5.5.

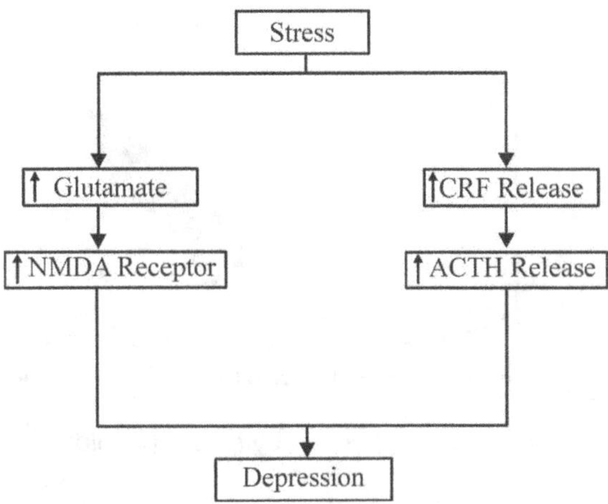

Figure 5.5 Pathophysiology of depression.

5.2.1 Experimental Models for Antidepressant Activity

(a) Despair swim test

Background: Porsolt et al. in 1977 described this experimental model. The animals are forced to swim in a restricted area from there they cannot escape. It causes induction of characteristics behavior of immobility along with assumption of floating posture. The behavior of animals causes a state of despair, which can be reduced by several clinically useful antidepressant drugs.

Requirements: Sprague-Dawley rats (150-180 g), plexiglass cylinder

Methodology

Selection of animals: Male Sprague-Dawley rats (150-180 g) are housed in individual polypropylene cages one day before the experiment, with free access to food and water.

Apparatus: The apparatus is made of glass, cylindrical shape with height 40 cm and diameter 18 cm, it contains 15 cm warm water [Figure 5.6].

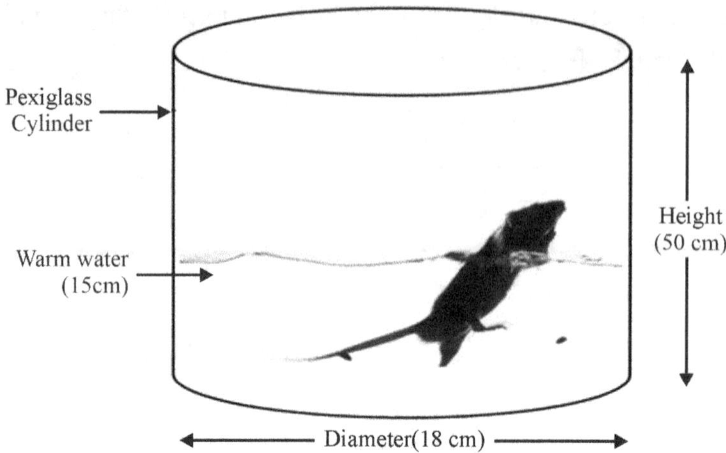

Figure 5.6 Induction of depression by placing in plexiglass cylinder.

Induction of depression: Following steps are taken to make animals depressive:

- The rats are allowed to swim in a cylinder.
- Animals, when placed first time in the cylinder are highly vigorous and active and try to climb the wall of the cylinder.
- Animal gets interspersed with the phases of increased immobility after 2-3 min of activity.
- The immobility reaches to plateau after 5-6 min at that the animal remain immobile for 80% of the time [Figure - 5.7].

Termination: Terminate the experiment after 15 min followed by removing animals from the cylinder and dry them at 32°C warm chamber and kept in their respective cages.

Repetition: The experiment repeated after 24 h by placing animals in the cylinder, the immobility duration is measured during a 5 min test.

Immobility: Immobility is achieved when animals remain floating passively on water in upright position, the nose just above the surface.

Administration: Both standard and test drugs are administered 1 h before testing.

Evaluation: Duration of immobility is recorded in control and in animals of the various treatment groups. Antidepressants significantly reduce the immobility and dose-responses can be evaluated.

Advantages:

- Relative simplicity is the significant advantage of this method.

- This method is effective for atypical antidepressants that are inactive in other classical tests.

Note: Rats are more suitable for screening antidepressant activity using this method.

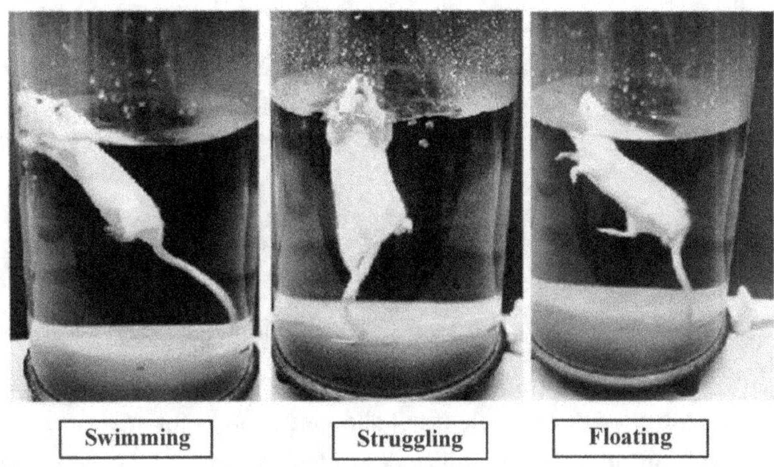

Figure 5.7 Forced swim test.

(b) Tail suspension test in mice

Background: Animals show immobility when they are subjected to escape stress that is not avoidable or escapable. It reflects despair behavior that indicates depressive disorder in humans. Antidepressant drugs reduce the immobility of animals that leads to active attempts of escaping while suspending them by the tail Figure 5.8.

Requirements: Mice (20-25 g), adhesive tape and table. 10 mice for each experimental group are taken.

Methodology

Acclimatization: Animals are acclimatized with the laboratory and environment for 10 days before commencement of experiment. They are provided with free access to water and food.

Administration of drug: Test drugs are given through intraperitoneal route 30 min before testing.

Induction of depression: Depression is induced by suspending animals on the edge of a shelf above a table top 58 cm above the ground with an adhesive tape from tip of the tail.

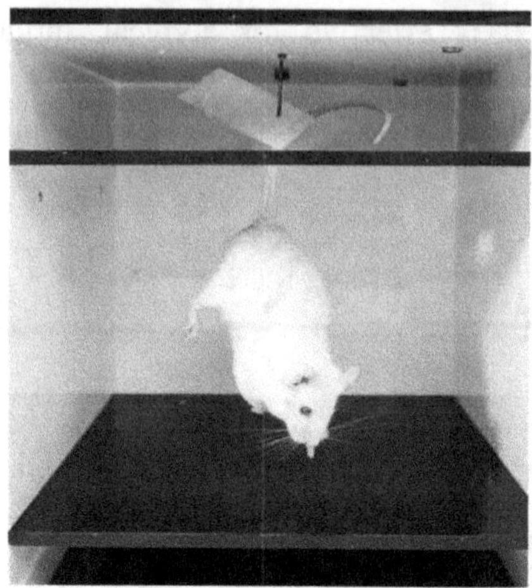

Figure 5.8 Tail suspension test in mice.

Recording: The immobility duration is noted for 5 min and animals are considered immobile if not showing motion for at least 60 sec.

Evaluation: The immobility percentage is counted and compared with control groups. The ED_{50} values of test compounds can be calculated.

Advantage: Tail suspension test is a facile means of screening the antidepressant drugs.

(c)   Learned helplessness in rats

Background: Sprague- Dawley rats are given a shock, and in training, there is no escape from it. This produces severe depression.

Methodology

Animals: Sprague- Dawley albino rats (150-220g)

Procedure: On exposure to electric shock for 60 min of about 0.7 mA for a schedule of 10s of shock per minute, the learned helplessness is produced in male Sprague-Dawley rats. The dimension of the apparatus used is 30×45×30 cm box with a grid floor. To allow a jump-up escape response, a platform is inserted about 7.5×7.5 cm through one side of the wall and at the height of 20 cm above the floor. During training, there is no platform. Using the same apparatus, the animals are tested for acquisition of jump-up escape after the appropriate treatment. While starting, an electric current is given by placing the platform into the box. The shock is terminated if animal do not escape from the platform within 10 s. However, if animal try to escape then they are allowcd to remain in the platform for 10 s and then returned to the grid floor. Ten such trials are performed on the interval on the 20s. This training helps in improving the learning behavior of 80% animals.

(d) Apomorphine induced hypothermia

Background: Apomorphine increases temperature in mice which is depressed by the antidepressant drug, and these drugs are well screened with the help of this model.

Requirement: Swiss mice (20-22 g), apomorphine.

Methodology

Procedure: Apomorphine (16 mg/kg, i.p) is administered after 60 min of test drug administration and body temperature of mice are monitored with a thermometer after 10, 20 and 30 min of apomorphine administration. A curve is constructed between time and temperature. The AUC is determined for all treated groups and then converted into percentage inhibition of apomorphine-induced hypothermia in comparison to control group. Linear regression curve is plotted to determine ED_{50}.

Advantages

- It is a very easy procedure to carry out.
- Simple and less time consuming.

5.3   Antiepileptic Activity

Epilepsy is the extraneuronal discharges in the brain that is characterized by cerebral dysrhythmia, episodic disturbances of consciousness and other sensory or psychiatric phenomenon.

5.3.1 Experimental Model for Antiepileptic Activity

(a) Electric shock induced seizures in rodents

Background: The test compounds protect animals from electric shock that is used for induction of grand mal epilepsy. The antiepileptic drugs suppress tonic hind limb extensions due to electric stimuli. This method is also called as the maximal electroshock seizure (MES).

Requirements: Swiss mice or Wistar rats, electro-convulsiometer.

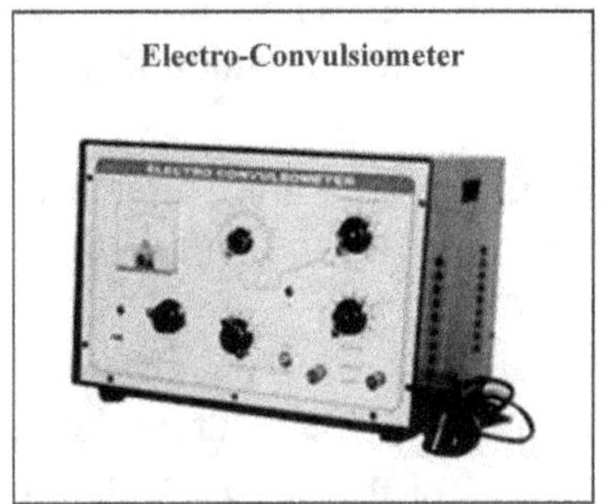

Figure 5.9 Electro-convulsiometer.

Methodology

Selection of animals: Swiss mice or Wistar rats weighing 20-32 g and 100-150 g respectively are used in the groups of 6-10 animals in each group.

Administration of drug: The test drug may be given by either intraperitoneal injection or orally.

Induction of convulsions: After 30 min of intraperitoneal injection or 60 min after oral administration the animals are subjected to electroshock.

An electro-convulsiometer [Figure 5.9] with corneal or ear electrodes is used to deliver the shock. The intensity of stimulus commonly employed is 12 mA, 50 Hz for 2 s for mice and 50 mA, 60 Hz for 2 s in rats.

Observation: The animals are observed for 2 min after the shock. The disappearance of the hind limb extensor tonic convulsions is taken as the criterion of protection.

Calculation: Percentage inhibition of seizures as compared to controls is calculated. Using different doses ED_{50} and 95% confidence intervals are calculated by probit analysis.

(b) Picrotoxin induced convulsions

Background: Picrotoxin is a GABA- antagonist, and it modifies the function of the chloride ion channel of the GABA receptor complex. Activation of GABA receptor effects inhibition of the post-synaptic cell by increasing the flow of chloride ions into the cells, which tends to hyperpolarize the neurons. Benzodiazepines are known to enhance GABA receptor mediated inhibition through distinct actions on the GABA receptor.

Requirements: Groups of 10 Swiss mice of either sex (20-25 g), diazepam, picrotoxin.

Methodology

Administration of drug: They are treated either orally or intraperitoneally with the test compound or standard (diazepam 10 mg/kg, i.p.).

Induction of convulsions: 30 min after i.p. or 60 min after oral administration of test and standard compounds the animals are injected with picrotoxin (3.5 mg/kg, s.c).

Observation: The animals are then observed for the symptoms of clonic and tonic seizures and death during the next 30 min.

Recording: Time taken for the onset of seizures and causing death are carefully recorded.

Calculation: ED_{50} values are calculated by using 3-4 doses of test and standard drugs and taking the percentage of seizures in the vehicle treated group as 100%.

(c) Pentylenetetrazol (Metrazol) induced convulsions

Background: Pentylenetetrazol is a useful laboratory tool for screening anticonvulsant drugs. It produces generalized synchronized chronic movements which are superseded by tonic convulsion characterized by flexion of limbs followed by the extension. This test is considered indicative of anticonvulsant activity of drugs against petit mal seizures [Figure 5.10].

Requirements: Swiss albino mice (20-32 g) or Wistar albino rats of either sex (120-150 g), metrazol.

Methodology

Administration of drug: The test compound and the standard drug are injected s.c or i.p or orally to groups of 6-10 animals.

Induction of epilepsy: Metrazol (60 mg/kg, s.c or orally (p.o) is administered 30 min after injection or 60 min after oral administration of test drug.

Observation: Each animal is placed into an individual propylene cage for observation lasting 60 min.

Recording: Seizures, tonic-clonic convulsions and time taken for the onset for seizures are recorded.

Evaluation: The number of protected animals in the treated groups is calculated as a percentage of animals showing seizures in the control group. ED_{50} values for the test and reference drugs are calculated for comparison.

Stages of Epilepsy

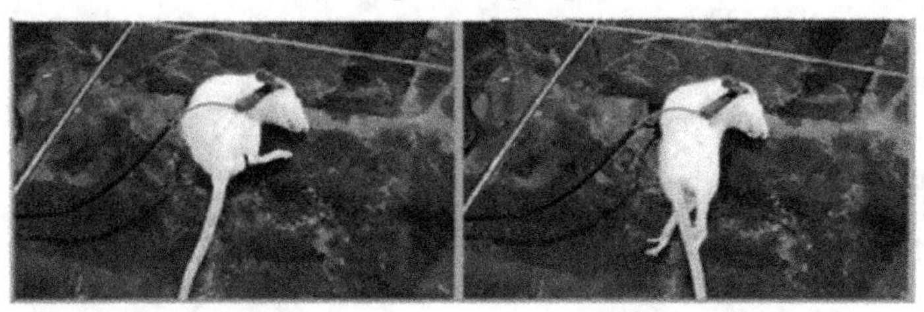

Figure 5.10 Pentylenetetrazol (metrazol) induced convulsions.

(d) Strychnine induced convulsion

Background: Strychnine produces tonic convulsion due to its glycine inhibiting activity. Anti convulsant drugs can be screened using this model.

Methodology: Mice (n=10) are used for this study. At first, they are treated with test or standard drug (orally), after 60 min, mice are injected with the strychnine nitrate (2 mg/kg, i.p.).

Observations: The behavior of the mice is observed for tonic convulsion and time of death is also noted. At this dose, convulsions are seen in 80 % of the animals.

Evaluation: ED_{50} values are calculated for various doses.

(e) Isoniazid induced convulsion

Background: Isoniazid inhibits GABAergic transmission and produces a tonic-clonic seizure in mice.

Methodology: 10 mice are used for this study, and they are administered with test or standard (diazepam-10mg/kg, i.p) and control group receive vehicle. After 30 min of i.p administration and 60 min of oral administration isoniazid (300 mg/kg, s.c) is administered.

Observation: clonic seizure, tonic seizure and death time are observed till 120 min.

(f) Yohimbine-induced convulsions

Background: Yohimbine induces a seizure in mice. Suppression of yohimbine induced convulsion is one of the right models to screen the GABA agonistic activity.

Procedure: Mice are placed in the plastic cylinder, and yohimbine is administered (45 mg/kg, s.c) after 30 min of test or standard compound.

Observation: The number of clonic seizures is observed for 60 min.

Evaluation: ED_{50} values are calculated.

5.4 Antipsychotic Activity

The dopamine hypothesis of schizophrenia, the defects in attention seen in patients with schizophrenia and the dopamine antagonist properties of psychoactive drugs, all lend themselves to animal model development. Animal models are divided into two broad categories viz. the behavioral tests and the tests based on pharmacological antagonism or the mechanism of action of antipsychotic drugs [Figure 5.11].

Experimental models for psychosis

5.4.1 Behavioral Test Models

(a) Innate behavior of golden hamsters

Background: Neuroleptic drugs reduce the aggressive behavior of male golden hamster in doses which do not impair motor function. This test can differentiate between neuroleptic and sedative/hypnotic activity.

Requirements: Golden hamsters, inclined board, glass jars.

Methodology:

Selection of animals: Golden hamsters (60-120 g, n=6) is used for performing the neuroleptic activity.

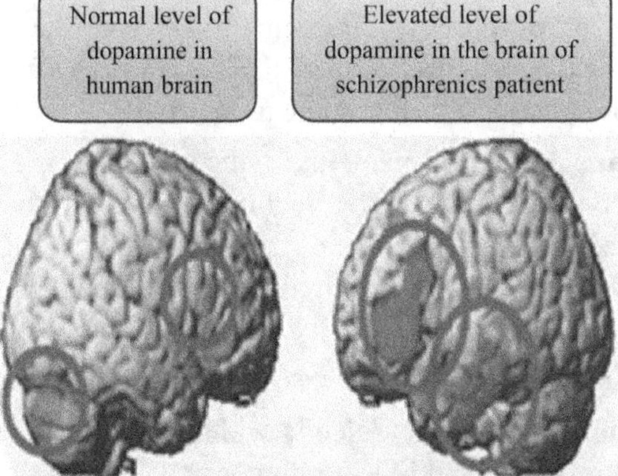

Figure 5.11 Dopamine hypothesis.

Acclimatization: 10-20 animals are placed together in crowded conditions in specially designed cages for at least 14 days. During this period these animals develop a typical fighting behavior.

Involvement of animals: Following steps are performed to include an animal in the study

- Animals are placed into a glass jar of 2 liters capacity.
- If they are held with a blunted forceps, an innate characteristic behavior is elicited.
- The hamster throws itself onto his back, tries to bite and to push the forceps away with his legs and utters angry shrieks.
- The animals are repeatedly touched in this way upto 6 times followed by punching with the forceps.
- Only those animals which respond to the stimuli with all three defense reactions, i.e. turning, vocalizing and biting are included in the test.

Administration of drug: The test compounds can be administered sub-cutaneously (s.c), intraperitoneally (i.p) or orally (p.o), 6 to 8 animals are used for each dose.

Stimulation: Stimuli are applied every 20 min for 3 h in the treated and control hamsters.

Condition of psychoses: The animals are considered fully 'tamed' when all the defense reactions are suppressed even after punching with the forceps at least once during the test period.

Treatment: After treatment, the tamed animals are placed on the inclined board with 20 degree inclination. The normal hamsters and drug treated hamsters are able to support themselves or to climb on the board. The hamsters with impaired motor function slide down.

Note: Animals motor function is considered disturbed if it falls three times during the two tests of the experiments.

Evaluation: The term neuroleptic width indicates the ration between the ED_{50} for taming and ED_{50} for motor impairment.

Advantages

- Neuroleptics can be easily differentiated from the sedative and hypnotic drugs.
- This method neither requires the training of the animals, nor there is a need for any expensive apparatus.

(b) Catalepsy in rats

Background: Catalepsy in rodents is induced by neuroleptic drugs. These drugs have an inhibitory effect on the nigrostriatal dopamine system. Cataleptic symptoms in rodents also indicate the potential of antipsychotic drugs for producing Parkinsonism like extrapyramidal side effects when used clinically.

Requirements: Wistar rats, wooden bars, stop watch

Methodology

Selection of animals: Groups of 6 male Wistar rats (150-200 g) are used.

Procedure: Test drug is given intraperitoneally. After 30 min animals are placed individually into translucent plastic boxes with a wooden dowel mounted horizontally 10 cm from the floor and 4 cm from the end to the box.

Induction of psychoses: The animals are allowed to adapt to the box for 5 min. Thereafter each animal is grasped gently around the shoulders and under the forepaws and placed carefully on the dowel.

Observation: The amount of time spent with at least one forepaw on the bar is noted down. When the animal removes its paws, the time is recorded, and the rat is repositioned on the bar. Four trials are conducted for each animal at 30, 60, 120 and 360 min. An animal is considered cataleptic if it remains on the bar for 60s.

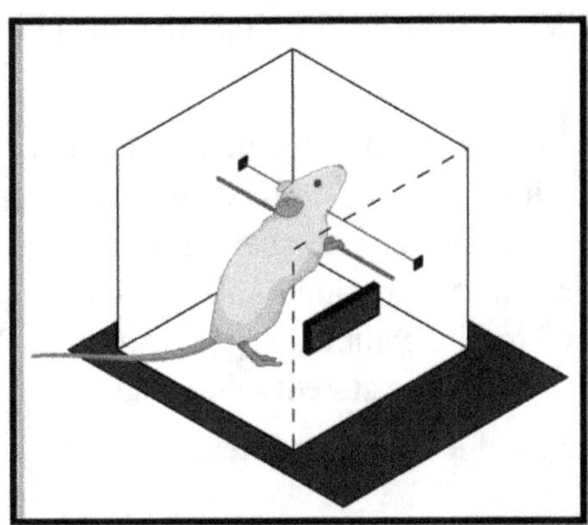

Figure 5.12 Catalepsy in rodents.

5.4.2 Tests Based on Pharmacologic Antagonism

(a) **Amphetamine group toxicity**

Background: The increased toxicity results from amphetamine administration leads to increased level of circulating catecholamines following aggregation which produces marked behavioral activation. After the administration of amphetamine in high doses, mice exhibit an elevated motor activity which is followed by death within 24 h in

80-100% of control animals. Neuroleptics reduces the death rate occurred due to amphetamine.

Requirements: Ten male Swiss mice (20-25 g), d-amphetamine

Methodology

Administration: Test or standard drugs given i.p or orally and placed in glass jars of 18 cm diameter.

Induction: 30 min after test drug administration, mice, receive 20 mg/kg of d-amphetamine s.c.

Observation: The mortality is then assessed at 1, 4 and 24 h after its administration. The mortality in control group is 80%.

Estimation: ED_{50} values are calculated for protection and their confidence limits are calculated.

Advantage: The amphetamine group toxicity has been rated as a reliable method for assessing neuroleptic activity.

(b) Amphetamine stereotypy in rats

Background: Amphetamine releases catecholamines and induces peculiar stereotypic behavior in rats.

Requirments: Wistar albino rats, amphetamine (10 mg/kg, s.c)

Methodology:

Procedure: SixWistar rats are injected with amphetamine (10 mg/kg; s.c) at the same time, and test or standard compound intraperitoneally and then they are placed in their respective cages. Stereotypic behavior, i.e. persistent repetition of an act is observed for 60 min such as sniffing, chewing, the compulsive gnawing, etc. The test compound may elevate or suppress the stereotypic behavior.

Evaluation: ED_{50} values are calculated.

5.5   Anti-Parkinsonian Activity

It is an extrapyramidal motor disorder characterized by rigidity, tremor, and hypokinesia with secondary manifestations like defective posture and gait, mask-like face and sialorrhoea; dementia may accompany. If left untreated the patient may be rigid, unable to move, unable to breathe properly and succumbs mostly to chest infection.

The most consistent lesion in Parkinson's disease (PD) is degeneration of neurons in the substantia nigra pars compacta (SN-PC) and nigrostriatal (dopaminergic) tract. This results in a deficiency of dopamine in the striatum which controls muscle tone and coordinates movements. A synthetic toxin N-methyl-4-phenyl tetrahydropyridine (MPTP), which occurs as a contaminant of some illicit drugs, produces nigrostriatal degeneration and manifestations similar to Parkinson's disease. Lesions of the nigrostriatal tract or chemically induced depletion of dopamine in the experimental animals also produce symptoms of PD. Rigidity and tremors involve more complex neurochemical disturbances of other transmitters particularly acetylcholine, 5-HT, NE and GABA as well as dopamine.

5.5.1 Experimental Models for Antiparkinsonian Drugs

(a) Tremorine and oxotremorine tremors

Background: These are centrally as well as peripherally acting cholinergic agents. They are known to induce Parkinsonism like signs and symptoms comprising of tremors, ataxia, spasticity, salivation, lacrimation, and hypothermia in rodents. These symptoms are prevented by centrally acting anticholinergic drugs, which have been used in the treatment of Parkinsonism for a long time.

Requirements: Swiss male mice (20-25 g, n=10), oxotremorine.

Methodology

Administration of drug: Test drug is administered 60 min prior to induction of Parkinsonism.

Induction of parkinsonian likes condition: by oxotremorine (0.5 mg/kg, s.c)

Temperature: Rectal temperature is measured before the administration of compound and 1, 2 and 3 h after oxotremorine injection.

Score: Tremors are scored in 10 s observation periods; every 15 min for 1 h. Salivation and lacrimation are also scored 15, and 30 min after oxotremorine injection and these symptoms are graded as given below:

Tremor, Salivation, and Lacrimation	Score
Absent	0
Slight	1
Moderate	2
Severe	3

Note: Hypothermia, tremor, salivation and lacrimation scores are recorded similarly, and the average values are statistically compared between test/standard and control groups.

(b) MPTP induced Parkinsonism in the monkeys

Background: MPTP (N-methyl-4-phenyl-1,2,3,6-tetrahydropyridine) causes irreversible destruction of nigrostriatal dopaminergic neurons in various species, and produces a PD like state in primates. MPTP acts by being converted to a toxic metabolite MPP^+ by the MAO-B subtype. MPP^+ is taken by the dopamine transport system, and thus acts selectively on the dopaminergic neurons; it inhibits mitochondrial oxidation reactions, producing oxidative stress.

Requirements: Rhesus monkey, MPTP (N-methyl-4-phenyl-1, 2, 3, 6-tetrahydropyridine)

Methodology

Selection of animals: Rhesus monkey (6-8 kg, n=10)

Induction of Parkinsonism: Treatment provided for 5-8 days with cumulative i.v doses of 10-18 mg/kg of MPTP.

Administration of drug: Symptoms of akinesia, rigidity, postural tremor, flexed posture, eyelid closure, and drooling are reversed by the treatment with levodopa.

Pathological changes: The pathological and biochemical changes are observed.

Scoring: The severity of parkinsonism can be scored as

Criteria	Scores				
	0	1	2	3	4
Tremors at rest	Absent	Slight and infrequently present	Mild in amplitude and persistent	Moderate in amplitude and present most of the time	Marked in amplitude and present most of the time
Facial expression	Normal	Minimal hypomimia	Slight but definitely abnormal diminution of facial expression	Moderate hypomimia	Masked or fixed facies with severe or complete loss of facial expression
Action or postural tremors	Absent	Slight; present with action	Moderate in amplitude, present with action	Moderate in amplitude with posture holding as well as action	Marked in amplitude; interferes with feeding
Rigidity	Absent	Slight	Mild to moderate	Marked, but full range of motion easily achieved	Severe, range of motion achieved with difficulty

Table *Contd...*

Criteria	Scores				
	0	**1**	**2**	**3**	**4**
Posture	Normal	Slightly stooped posture	Moderately stooped posture	Severely stooped posture with kyphosis	Marked flexion with extreme abnormality of posture
Gait	Normal	Walks slowly	Walks with difficulty	Severe disturbance of gait	Cannot walk at all
Body bradykinesia and hypokinesia	None	Minimal slowness	Mild degree of slowness	Moderate slowness	Marked slowness

(c) Reserpine antagonism

Background: Reserpine depletes the central catecholamine stores and other biogenic amines like 5-HT etc. It produces marked sedation in mice along with hypokinesia, rigidity, and immobility. These effects are antagonized by reserpine antagonist and used for the treatment of Parkinsonism.

Requirements: Swiss mice (20-25 g, either sex), reserpine, perspex cages.

Methodology

Procedure: Reserpine (5 mg/kg, i.p) is administered 24 h before the test compound administration. The test compounds and standard drug are administered 30 min before recording the observations.

Performance of test: The animals are then placed individually in Perspex cages (30 × 26 × 20 cm).

Recording: Horizontal movements, rearing, and grooming episodes are recorded for 10 min.

Evaluation: The locomotor activity and grooming scores of control and treated animals are noted and compared.

References

- Gupta, S. K., 2004. Drug screening methods. Jaypee brothers medical publishers LTD. New Delhi. pp. 61-117.
- Lawrence, D. R., Bucharach, A. L., 1684. Evaluation of drug activities: Pharmacometrics. Academic press, London and New York. pp. 897.

- Papa SM, Chase TN. Levodopa-induced dyskinesias improved by a glutamate antagonist in Parkinsonian monkeys. Ann Neurol 1996; 39(5): 574-8.

- Tripathi, K.D., 2003. Essential of medical pharmacology. Jaypee brothers medical publishers. New Delhi. pp. 167-184.

- Turner, A. R., 1965.Screening methods in pharmacology. Academic press New York and London. pp. 69-82.

- Vogel, H.G., 2002. Drug Discovery and evaluation: Pharmacological assays. Springer-verlag berlin Heidelberg publication. New York, pp. 1-15.

Chapter 6

Evaluation of Drugs Acting on Respiratory System

6.1 Bronchodilator and Anti-Asthmatic Activity

Asthma is a chronic and severe lung disease that constricts the airways. It is a syndrome that causes a reversible obstruction of airways to external stimuli. Asthma leads to chest tightness, wheezing, coughing and shortness of breath. Symptoms of asthma is mainly seen in night and early morning. In asthmatic patient there are increased inflammatory reactions and inflammatory mediators like eosinophills, leukotrienes etc. The models for testing efficacy of antiasthmatic drugs have been used extensively to determine the mechanism of drug. However, the mechanism of disease is still unclear.

Genetic and environmental factors are responsible for development of asthma, it may also provoke allergic reactions and obstruction of airways. Allergic reactions may occur due to pollution, mites, house dust, pet dander, pollens, chemical irritants, tobacco smoke, etc. Other provoking factors for asthma are cold air, anger, heavy exercise and drugs (aspirin and beta blockers).

6.1.1 *In Vitro* Methods

(a) **Spasmolytic activity on guinea pigs isolated tracheal chain**

Background: The tracheal chain is separated from guinea pigs. They are used for testing compounds which inhibit bronchospasm. It detects β sympathomimetics, H_1-receptor antagonist and leukotriene blocking properties of the test drugs.

Requirements: Male guinea pigs (250-400 g), anesthetics, Krebs-Henseleit solution, histamine or carbachol, aminophylline.

Methodology

Procedure: Animals are sacrificed using inhalational anesthetics. Slices of removed trachea is done as individual ring and tied with thread to mount on the organ bath using Krebs-Henseleit solution. The assembly is maintained at 37 °C temperature with tension of 0.5 g, it is gassed with carbogen. Isometric contractions are recorded via a strain gauge transducer on a polygraph. Forty five minutes are allowed for equilibration before the addition of spasmogen. Spasmogens like histamine or carbachol are used in the concentration of 10^{-7} and 2×10^{7} g/ml respectively. After 10-12 min for reaching the contraction to a maximum the test drugs (e.g. aminophylline, 10 mg/ml) are administered. The bronchial response is recorded.

Evaluation: The percent inhibition of spasmogen induced contractions is calculated. ED_{50} is calculated, from the dose response curve.

6.1.2 *In Vivo* Methods

(a) Spasmolytic activity of Bronchioles in anaesthetized guinea pigs (Konzett-Rossler method)

Background: This method was given by Konzett and Rossler. It is based on measuring the volume of air changes in trachea and bronchi of animals in a closed chamber using respiratory pump. A reservoir is attached to the system for measuring pressure or volume of excess air. Spasm of bronchioles reduces the volume of inhaled air.

Requirements: Guinea pigs (250-400 g), urethane, respiratory pump, transducer, spasmogens (histamine), two way cannula, substance P, ovalbumin, leukotrienes, platelet activating factor

Methodology

Anaesthesia: Animals are anaesthetized with urethane (1.25 g/kg, i.p).

Cannulation: Trachea is cannulated by means of a two way cannula, one arm of which is connected to a respiratory pump and other to a transducer.

Artificial respiration: The animal is artificially respired using a Starling respiratory pump with an inspiratory pressure set at 90–120 mm of water, an adequate tidal volume of 3 ml/100 g body weight and a frequency of 60 strokes per min.

Induction of bronchospasm: Various spasmogens like histamine (5-20 µg/kg), substance P (0.5 µg/kg), ovalbumin (1 mg/kg), leukotrienes (25-50 µg/kg) and platelet activating factor (PAF, 25-50 µg/kg) can be used for producing bronchoconstriction.

Administration of drug: After obtaining two bronchospasms of equal intensity, test compounds are administered by the i.v. or s.c. and the spasmogen is repeated at 15, 30 and 60 min after the drug administration.

Calculation: The results are expressed as percent inhibition of induced bronchospasm over the control agonistic response and ED_{50} can be calculated by using graded doses of test drugs.

6.1.3 Bronchial Hyperactivity

Hyperactivity of bronchioles is measured as symptoms of asphyctic convulsions due to administration of antigens, histamine or other spasmogens. These symptoms may increase inspiration, breathing frequency, and anaphylactic convulsions. It can be delayed by the administration of antagonistic drugs.

(a) Histamine induced bronchial hyperactivity in guinea pigs

Background: Histamine induces asphyctic convulsion in guinea pigs which is similar with asthmatic attack.

Requirement: Guinea pigs (300-400 g), three boxes, histamine.

Procedure: Three boxes, box A, box B, box C are taken and they are supplied with aerosols. In box A guinea pig is placed and test or standard drug (0.2 ml/min) is administered using an ultrasound nebulizer then the animal is passed to box B (only air flow 1.5l/min) and finally the animal is made to go to box C and here the animal is exposed to histamine aerosol (0.1% solution). Time is noted down for asphyctic convulsion and the animal is removed from the box as soon as possible. ED_{50} (50% increase in preconvulsive time) is also calculated.

(b) Arthus type immediate hypersensitivity in rats

Background: The inflammatory symptoms is seen in rheumatoid arthritis patients. It is due to activation of polymorphonuclear neutrophils (PMNs) and complement system due to antigen-antibody reactions. It leads to inflammation that is characterized by vasculitis, haemorrhage, and oedema.

Requirements: Wistar or Sprague Dawley albino rats (150-200 g), ovalbumin-Pertusis vaccine suspension (ovalbumin, paraffin oil, 0.9% saline solution, pertussis vaccine), plethysmometer.

Methodology:

Sensitization of animals: Seven days prior to experiment, these animals are sensitized by i.m administration of 0.5 ml of albumin-pertusis vaccine suspension.

Note: Ovalbumin suspension is prepared by suspending 1700 mg of ovalbumin in 100 ml of paraffin oil. Then 4.38 ml of pertussis vaccine is suspended in 70 ml of 0.9% saline solution. Both these suspensions are mixed to form an emulsion.

Arrangement: Animals are allowed standard chow diet and water *ad libitum* 24 h and 60 min prior to the induction of arthus reaction.

Administration of test drug: Test drug is given to sensitized rats through suitable route.

Induction of arthus reaction: 0.1 ml of 0.04% of ovalbumin by subplantar injection in left paw causes swelling of paw within hours.

Measurement: Paw volume is measured by plethymometric method.

Evaluation: Percent reduction in paw volume shows the effectiveness of drug.

6.2   Antitussive Activity

6.2.1 Experimental Model of Antitussive Drugs

(a) Citric acid inhalation induced cough in guinea pigs

Background: Production of cough is a reflex action. The receptors, which are sensitive to various types of stimuli leading to cough, are located in the bronchial pathway, mostly in the region where the trachea bifurcates. These receptors are activated either mechanically or chemically i.e. by inhalation of various irritants. The nerve impulses in turn activate the cough centre in the brain. The most commonly used method for producing cough is through the inhalation of citric acid aerosol in guinea pigs.

Requirements: Guinea pigs (300-350 g, either sex), cylindrical glass, 7.5 % citric acid, citric acid aerosol

Methodology

Chamber: The animal is placed in a specially designed cylindrical glass vessel which has two tubes at either ends. Through one of them the aerosol is sprayed and other is meant for its efflux.

Recorder: The efflux tube has a side arm connected to a tambour through which the pressure changes can be recorded. The displacement in the air caused by coughing of the animal is recorded.

Exposure: The guinea pig is then exposed to an aerosol of 7.5 % citric acid in water for 10 min.

Administration of drug: After one hour the test drug is administered either orally or s.c. and 30 min later the animal is again exposed to citric acid aerosol and the number of tussal responses are recorded during 10 min.

Calculation: The number of coughs after treatment with test/standard drugs is expressed as percentages of the control period. Using graded doses the ED_{50} values can be calculated.

Note: This method has been widely used for screening of antitussive drugs and is known to produce reproducible and dependable results.

(b) Mechanical stimulation induced cough in guinea pigs

Background: Mechanical stimulation in anaesthetized guinea pigs can lead to production of severe cough which responds to drugs like codeine in a dose dependent manner.

Requirements: Guinea pigs (300-350 g, either sex), 25 % urethane, heating plate, steel wire, codeine sulphate. Minimum of 10 animals are used as controls and for each dose of test and standard drug.

Methodology

Acclimatization: Animals are acclimatized at least one week before the experiment and maintained in standardized conditions at 21 ± 2 °C, relative humidity 55 ± 10 % and at 12 hour on 12 hour off light cycle with food and water given *ad libitum*.

Anaesthesia: The animals are anaesthetized with 25 % urethane (4 ml/kg, i.p).

Temperature: The body temperature of guinea pigs is maintained constantly at 37 °C by means of a heated plate.

Incision: Trachea is incised by inserting thin steel wire near the carotid cartilage. While pushing the wire inside it causes production of cough by reaching the bifurcation of the trachea. The induction is performed at 5 min prior to oral drug administration and 30, 60 and 120 min after treatment.

Administration of drug: The animals which respond to both the stimulations before the administration of drugs are selected and then randomly assigned to receive either the test drug or a standard drug (Codeine sulphate: 15, 30 and 60 mg/kg).

Calculation: The results are subjected to the evaluation of statistical significance by Student's-t-test for paired data and ED_{50} values are determined.

6.3   Expectorant Activity

(a) Acute study of mucus secretion in rabbits

Background: This method was given by Perry and Boyd (1941) based on collecting bronchial mucus from rabbits. Respiratory tract disorders can produce both qualitative and quantitative changes in the mucus which covers and protects the airway epithelium. Methods of collecting the mucus from the bronchial tree are necessary for studying the effect of drugs.

Requirements: New Zealand rabbits of either sex (3-3.5 kg), urethane, T cannula, inclined board, centrifuge tubes, pilocarpine, ammonium chloride

Methodology

Anaesthesia: Animals are anaesthetized with urethane (1.2-1.4 g/kg, i.p.).

The trachea is opened to some extent about 2 cm below the carotid cartilage. One arm of a T cannula is placed inside the trachea which is connected to an air outlet of a humidifier (temperature 37-38 °C, relative humidity 80 %). The other arm is joined to collection tube. The rabbit is then restrained in the supine position on a 60° inclined board with the head downwards. Fluid from respiratory tract is collected in centrifuge tubes at intervals of 60 min. The secretion of mucus can be induced by vagal stimulation or by ammonium chloride given by stomach tube or pilocarpine administered intraperitoneally.

Calculation: Time response curves after the stimulants of mucus secretion are compared with that of control animals.

(b) Bronchoalveolar lavage in guinea pigs

Background: This method is based on the isolation of bronchial cells from bronchoalveolar lavage in anaesthetized guinea pigs.

Requirements: Guinea pigs (300-350 g, either sex), pentobarbitone sodium, phosphate buffer saline, EDTA, isoproterenol.

Methodology:

Anaesthesia: Animals are anaesthetized using 70 mg/kg of pentobarbitone sodium intraperitoneal.

Cannulation: The trachea, jugular vein and carotid artery are exposed and cannulated.

Lavage: After adjusting all mechanical respiratory parameters, the bronchoalveolar lavage is performed through the tracheal cannula. The lungs are lavaged with 5 aliquots of 10 ml phosphate buffered saline containing 3 mM EDTA and 100 µm isoproteronol (pH 7.2-7.4).

Centrifugation: The recovered lavage fluid (40-45 ml) is centrifuged, the cells are re-suspended in 20 ml of phosphate-buffered saline and the total cells are counted using a hemocytometer. The remaining aliquot is centrifuged again and the cells are stained to determine the differential cell count.

Calculation: The differences in cells recovered from bronchoalveolar lavage between treatments groups are tested by the use of one way analysis of variance.

References

- Holmes, A. M., Solari, R., Holgate, S.T. Animal models of asthma: value, limitations and opportunities for alternative approaches.Drug Discov.Today. 2011; 16, 659-670.

- Patel, K. N., Chorawala, M. R. Animal Models of asthma. Journal of Pharmaceutical Research and Opinion. 2011; 1(5):139 - 147.

- Shin, Y. S., Takeda, K., Gelfand, E. W. Understanding asthma using animal models. Allergy Asthma Immunology Research. 2009; 1(1): 10-18.

- Gupta, S. K. Drug screening methods. Jaypee brothers medical publishers LTD. New Delhi.2004; 37-44.

Chapter 7

Evaluation of Drugs Acting on Eye

7.1 Anti-Cataract Activity

Cataract is leading cause of blindness worldwide. There are three types of cataract.

- **Nuclear cataract**: Nuclear cataract occurs in the centre of the lens. It is mostly seen in case with ageing.

- **Cortical cataract:** Cortical cataract progression starts from outside of the lens to the center of the eye.

- **Sub- capsular cataract:** This sub-capsular cataract starts from back of the lens and seen as a small opacity within the capsule. Figure 7.1 depicts about normal and cataractous lens of rats.

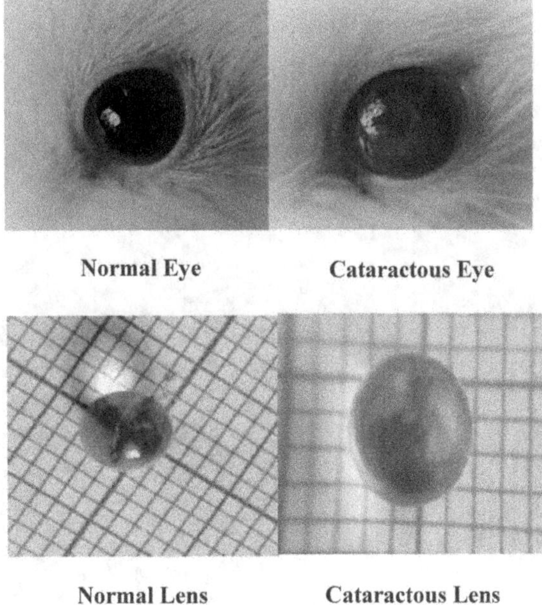

Figure 7.1 Normal and Cataractous lens of rat.

***In Vitro* Models**

H_2O_2 induced model, Rat Lens Organ Culture, Glucose induced model

***In Vivo* Models**

Galactose induced model, Alloxan induced cataract, Streptozotocin induced diabetic cataract, Selenite induced cataract and hypertension induced cataract.

7.1.1 *In Vitro* Models

(a) H_2O_2 induced models

Background: H_2O_2 is a non-radical member of active oxygen and is toxic to the lens. Active oxygen species cause peroxidation of lipids and lens proteins and thus increases cataractogenesis.

Requirements: Goat lenses, H_2O_2, TC 199

Methodology: Goat lenses are removed from the eyeballs by intracapsular lens extraction method within one hour of the death of the animal. Lenses are incubated individually in TC-199 media for 72 h. The medium is supplemented with 30% H_2O_2 solution at the final concentration of 10mM. This method induces cataract in goat lenses which can be observed by photographic methods [Figure 7.2]. Various stages of cataract are graded as:

Stage 0: Same like normal lens

Stage I: Faint peripheral opacity

Stage II: Irregular peripheral opacity

Stage III: Faint opalescence visible with naked eye

Stage IV: Mature nuclear cataract

Stage V: Opacity involving entire lens

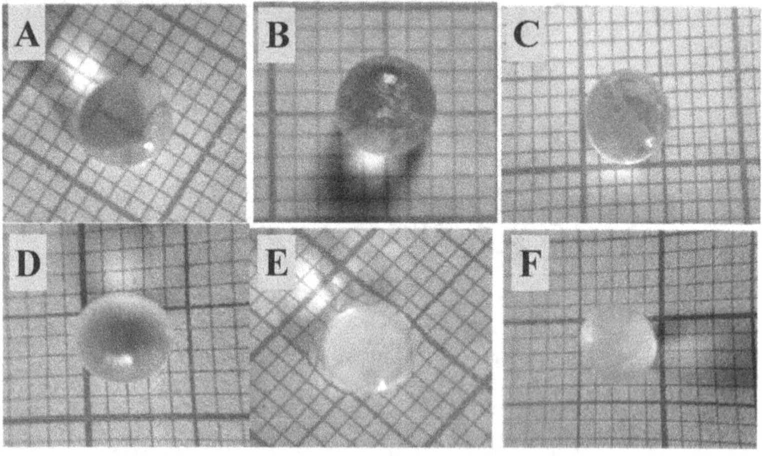

Figure 7.2 Stages of cataract formation. A, B, C, D, E and F indicating stage 0, I, II, III, IV and V respectively.

(b) Rat lens organ culture

Background: This model is used to screen the anti- cataract drugs.

Requirements: Rat lens, TC-199, H_2O_2

Methodology: The rats are sacrificed by asphyxiation with CO_2 or other recommended methods. Lenses are removed from the eye. The lenses are placed individually in a 24-well plate, incubated in TC-199 medium and in the presence of 0.5 mM H_2O_2 for 24 hours to induce cataract and then replaced with fresh H_2O_2 free medium for another 24 hour for recovery. Stages of cataract can be graded as discussed under H_2O_2 induced model.

(c) Glucose induced model

Background: Polyol pathway is related to the reduction of glucose to sorbitol due to activation of aldose reductase (AR) enzyme. This process is directly linked with the diabetic cataract. Liquefaction of lens fibers occur due to accumulation of polyols that leads to the lens opacity.

Requirements: rat lens, glucose

Methodology

From pairs of rat lenses, one lens is kept in medium with 55.6 mM glucose (10 times the normal concentration in the medium), while the other lens is kept in medium with a normal (5.56 mM) glucose concentration. The high concentration of glucose induces cataract. Lower concentrations are unsuitable in this model since they prolong the time of cataract development. The osmolarities of the high and normal glucose media are 348 and 306 mosm /kg, respectively. All lenses are incubated at 37°C with humidity of 95% air /5% CO_2 in 24-well culture plates and the culture medium changed daily.Stages of cataract can be graded as discussed under H_2O_2 induced model.

7.1.2 *In Vivo* Models

(a) Galactose induced cataract model

Background: High sugar intake can increase the risk of cataract formation. This model is used to screen anti-cataract agents.

Requirements: Albino rats (130-180g), Galactose

Methodology: Animals are given 30% galactose in their diet. They are also provided with free access of water and diet. The rats are divided into control and treatment group. Various test agents to be screened are administered to the treatment group. Eyes are examined by a portable hand-held slit lamp biomicroscope to detect the lens opacity after every 3 days. After 3 weeks opacity in the lens is clearly visible to naked eyes. Stages of cataract can be graded as discussed under H_2O_2 induced model.

(b) Alloxan induced cataract model

Background: Alloxan is very toxic glucose analogue which accumulate in pancreatic β cells. Alloxan produces reactive oxygen species and causes death of pancreatic β cells.

Requirements: Albino rats (150-200g), alloxan

Methodology: Animals are administered with single intraperitoneal (i.p.) injection of alloxan (90 mg/kg) or subcutaneous injection of alloxan 100-175 mg/kg. After 3 days blood glucose level is checked. Diabetic animals are used for further study. After 12 week changes in the lens are observed. Stages of cataract can be graded as discussed under H_2O_2 induced model.

(c) Streptozotocin induced diabetic cataract model

Background: Streptozotocin is an antibiotic. At a dose of 60-70 mg/kg, it induces cataract. This model is most widely used method to induce diabetic cataract.

Requirements: Sprague-Dawley albino rats (130-180 g).

Methodology

Streptozotocin is dissolved in sodium citrate 0.02M buffer solution maintained at pH 5. Animals are administered with single dose of streptozotocin (60-70mg/kg; i.p.). Diabetes is induced after 3 days which is measured with glucometer. Diabetic animals are treated with different drugs. After 12 weeks cataractous changes are observed. Various anti-cataract agents can be screened with this model. Stages of cataract can be graded as discussed under H_2O_2 induced model.

(d) Selenite induced cataract model

Background: This model is used to screen anti-cataract agents. Selenite produces bilateral nuclear cataract.

Requirements: Sprague-Dawley albino rats (130-180 g), selenite.

Methodology: Cataract is induced by single administration of sodium selenite (19-30μmoles/kg) through subcutaneous route generally in pups. After 16 days cataractous changes are observed. Frequent administration of smaller dose of selenite also produces cataract or sometimes oral route can also produce cataract. Stages of cataract can be graded as discussed under H_2O_2 induced model.

(e) Fructose induced hypertensive cataract model

Background: Blood pressure increases due to increased dietary intake of carbohydrates that leads to development of hypertension induced cataract.

Requirement: Wistar or Sprague Dawley albino rats (130-180 g) and fructose.

Methodology: Hypertension is induced in animals by giving high carbohydrate diet i.e. fructose solution (10%, w/v) in the drinking water for six weeks. Blood pressure increase is monitored from third week onwards. It can be checked by non-invasive blood pressure instrument (NIBP).The animals treated with test compounds from week four to six. The eyes and BP of animals are monitored regularly during the experiment. The animals are sacrificed after experiment and eyeballs are removed followed by separation of both lenses. Stages of the cataract can be graded as discussed under H_2O_2 induced model. Blood is collected from animals through cardiac puncture for analysis. Serum is also separated from blood and stored at cold temperature for various cataractogenic parameters. Biochemical parameters like glucose level, oxidative stress markers, lipid peroxidation and inflammatory mediators are estimated.

(f) Cadmium chloride ($CdCl_2$) induced hypertension

Background: The role of cadmium in hypertension has been considered for the past two decades. It is reported that chronic administration of the Cadmium chloride ($CdCl_2$) to albino rats significantly induces hypertension and exacerbates lenticular opacity.

Requirement: Wistar or Sprague Dawley albino rats (130-180 g) and fructose.

Methodology: Hypertension is induced in animals by giving $CdCl_2$ (0.5 mg/kg/day, i.p.) for six weeks. Increase in blood pressure is monitored from third week onwards. It can be checked by non-invasive blood pressure instrument (NIBP).The animals treated with test compounds from week four to six. The eyes and BP of animals are monitored regularly during the experiment. The animals are sacrificed after experiment and eyeballs are removed followed by separation of both lenses. Stages of the cataract can be graded as discussed under H_2O_2 induced model. Blood from animals are collected through cardiac puncture for analysis and serum is separated from collected blood samples and stored at cold temperature for biochemical estimation like glucose level, oxidative stress markers, lipid peroxidation and inflammatory mediators.

(g) Two kidney one clip induced hypertensive cataract model (2K1C) model

Background: Clamped renal artery for 4 hr induces acute renal hypertension. This model is used to screen antihypertensive drugs. It is reported that 2K1C surgery significantly induces hypertension as well as exacerbates cataract.

Requirement: Wistar or Sprague Dawley albino rats (130-180 g), ketamine and xylazine.

Methodology: Animals are anaesthetized with ketamine and xylazine (60:10 mg/kg, i.p.). Renal artery is occluded for 4 h by placing a PVC coated clip into left hilum of the kidney and fixed into back muscles. The trachea is cannulated to facilitate spontaneous respiration and jugular vein in cannulated for the administration of test compounds. Renal arterial clip is removed which leads to rise in blood pressure due to elevated plasma renin level. All uninephrectomized animals are given 0.9% NaCl in the drinking water for six consecutive weeks. Blood pressure is checked by NIBP instrument. After induction of hypertension, from the beginning of fourth week until the end of sixth week, animals are treated with the test compound. During the experimental protocol eyes of the animals and blood pressure is checked biweekly. After completion of the experimental protocol animals are sacrificed and their eyeballs are removed. Both lenses are separated from the eye balls via posterior approach. Stages of the cataract can be graded as discussed under H_2O_2 induced model. Blood samples from animals are collected by the cardiac puncture, and serum is separated and stored at 2 - 8°C. Pathophysiological parameters like glucose level, oxidative stress markers, lipid peroxidation, and inflammatory mediators in serum and eye lenses are evaluated.

7.2   Anti Glaucoma Activity

Glaucoma is a progressive optic neuropathy. Glaucoma is characterized by damage of optic nerve with loss of visual function. It is associated with increased intraocular pressure Figure 7.3 depicts about normal and glaucomatous retina. There are various models which are used to screen anti-glaucoma drugs.

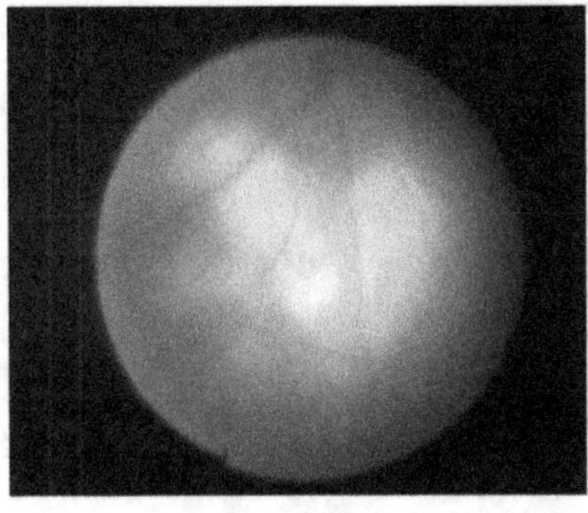

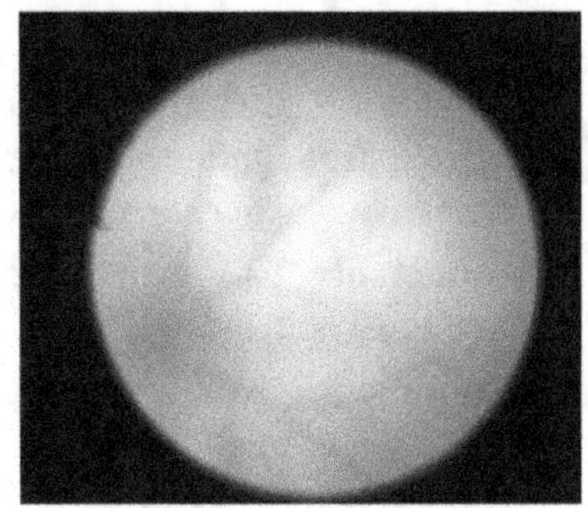

Figure 7.3 Normal and Glaucomatous retina of rat.

7.2.1 Experimental Animal Model for Anti Glaucoma Activity

(a) Intracameral injection of hyaluronic acid in the rats

Background: The cellular events of ganglionic cell death can be best understand using pressure-induced optic nerve damage of experimental mode. It occurs due to intraocular pressure and glaucoma.

Requirement: Male Wistar or Sprague Dawley rats (130-180 g), hyaluronic acid, ketamine.

Methodology: Animals are acclimatized to the laboratory condition prior the experiment with free access to food and water. Hyaluronic acid is given to animals once in a week on anterior chamber of the eye, however, saline is given to other eye. Ketamine hydrochloride (50 mg/ kg) and xylazine hydrochloride (0.5 mg/ kg) is given intraperitonealy to anesthetize the rats. Eyes are focused under a microscope (binocular Colden surgical) with coaxial light. Corneoscleral limbus region of the anterior chamber is focused through needle. The liquid progressively increase the chamber's depth with the help of bevel when it reaches towards the anterior chamber. Then separate the needle and avoid contact. The injection is given at corneoscleral limbus for 12 h and further injections is given by changing the head position for corneoscleral limbus. It is assessed by giving one drop of 0.5% proparacaine hydrochloride to each eye. Corneal edema is produced in most of the animals.

(b) Dexamethasone rat model of glaucoma

Background: Corticosteroid increases intraocular pressure. Dexamethasone induces ocular hypertension in ocular hypotensive and normotensive experimental animals.

Requirments: Wistar or Sprague Dawley rats (140-180 g, either sex), Dexamethasone and saline.

Methodology: Adult Wistar or Sprague Dawley rats (140-180 g, either sex) are maintained and trained to accept tonometry. During the baseline reading before the dexamethasone treatment, there is no significant difference between the IOP of the left and right eye. No signs of ocular irritation or inflammation are present. IOP is measured prior to and during all treatments after corneal anesthesia by topical application of proparacaine hydrochloride 0.5%. IOP is measured preferably at the same time and same interval during the experimental period. Dexamethasone sodium phosphate solution is diluted to the desired concentration of 0.5% or 1% with normal saline. This solution is applied to the corneal surface in a volume of 10μl with an automatic micropipette either unilaterally or bilaterally, one, two or three times daily. A gradual IOP increase is observed which becomes significant within 2 or 3 weeks.

7.3 Retinopathy

Progressive loss of vision and damage to retina can be defined as retinopathy. Diabetic retinopathy has following stages i.e. nonproliferative, pre-proliferative and proliferative. The main indicating factor of retinopathy in humans is total glycaemic exposure over time. The risk factors associated with retinopathy are renal disease, hypertension, tobacco consumption, pregnancy, and alcohol consumption. The pathways involved in the formation and progression of retinopathy are non-enzymatic glycation, polyol pathway and protein kinase C (PKC) activation due to oxidative damage of diacylglycerol (DAG). Figure 7.4 depicts about Normal Retina and Retinopathy.

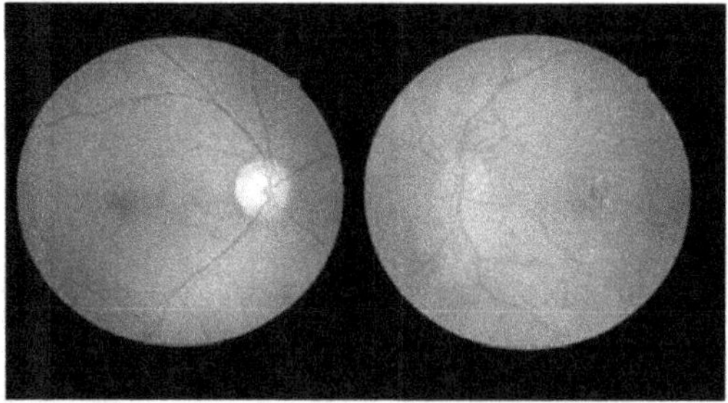

Figure 7.4 Normal Retina and Retinopathy in rat.

7.3.1 Experimental Animal Models for Retinopathy

(a) Diabetes induced retinopathy in rats

Background: In diabetic rats early stage lesions of retinopathy is clearly seen.

Requirements: BioBreeding (BB) rat, streptozotocin.

Methodology: Early changes in retinal function is best studied is BB rats along with the study of biochemical changes. Streptozotocin (STZ) induced rats show microangiopathic lesions (i.e. capillary basement thickening). Both types of animals models has been used in the study of abnormalities like blood flow to retina, electrophysiological changes in retina and permeability of membranes. Diabetes is induced by injection of STZ (65 mg/kg, i.p). Glucose is measured after one week in animals and high glucose level in animals is considered as diabetic.

(b) Galactosemic animal model

Background: Increased blood glucose level leads to development of diabetic retinopathy and other diabetes like complications like lesions in non-diabetic and hyperhexosemic animal models.

Requirment: Wistar or Sprague Dawley rats (140-180 g, either sex), galactose.

Methodology: The animals that are most often utilized in galactosemic studies are dogs and rats. Galactosemic rats were first developed to study the augmented polyol pathway. Early microangiopathic changes and micro-aneurysms are produced in this model. The isolation of raised hexose levels from other abnormalities of diabetes has given impetus to the argument for the importance of a polyol pathway in the pathogenesis of diabetic retinopathy. Continuation of galactose exposure results in the disease progression for the longer period of time, for example rats can be kept on high galactose diet for over 2 years. Retinal changes observed in the animals on a continuous high galactose diet include acellular capillaries and capillary basement membrane thickening.

References

- Kyselova, Z.Different experimental approaches in modelling cataractogenesis An overview of selenite-induced nuclear cataract in rats. Interdiscip Toxicol. 2010; 3(1): 3-14.

- Engerman, R. L., Kern, T. S. Hyperglycemia as a cause of diabetic retinopathy. Metabolism. 1986; 35(4):20-3.

- Khan, S. A., Choudhary, R., Singh A., Bodakhe, S. H. Hypertension potentiates cataractogenesis in rat eye through modulation of oxidative stress and electrolyte homeostasis. J. Curr. Ophthalmol. 28 (3) (2016) 123–130.

- Singh A., Khan, S. A., Choudhary, R., Bodakhe, S. H. Cinnamaldehyde attenuates cataractogenesis via restoration of hypertension and oxidative stress in fructosefed hypertensive rats. J. Pharmacopuncture. 19 (2) (2016) 137–144.

- Shrivastava, P., Choudhary, R., Nirmalkar, U., Singh, A., Shree, J., Vishwakarma, P.K., Bodakhe, S. H. Magnesium taurate attenuates progression of hypertension and cardiotoxicity against cadmium chloride-induced hypertensive albino rats. JTCM. 2017, 1-5.

- Shree J., Choudhary, R., Bodakhe S.H.. Losartan delays the progression of streptozotocin-induced diabetic cataracts in albino rats. Journal of Biochemistry and Molecular Toxicology. DOI: 10.1002/jbt.22342 ISSN: 1099-0461.

Chapter 8

Evaluation of Drugs Acting on Cardiovascular System

8.1 Antiarrhythmic Activity

An arrhythmia is an irregular heart beat. Normal heart rate is about 75 beats per minute. An atrial arrhythmia is deviation in the heart rate in any of the two upper chambers of the heart, the left or right atrium. A ventricular arrhythmia is irregularity produced in one of the two lower chambers of the heart, the left or right ventricle.

- **Atrial fibrillation:** It is an irregular heart rate characterized by rapid and irregular whipping.

- **Ventricular fibrillation:** Ventricular fibrillation is an in-coordination of ventricles contraction that causes vibration of cardiac muscles rather than contract properly. It is the most identified arrhythmia recorded during cardiac arrest.

- **Ventricular extra systoles:** Ventricular extra systoles are the extra beats that record during interruption of normal rhythm. The extra systoles record when the electrical discharge originates from somewhere other than sino-auricular node. It occurs after myocardial infarction.

- **Ventricular tachycardia:** Ventricular tachycardia is a malfunction of ventricles of heart due to very fast heartbeat when pulse rate increases more than 100 beast/min.

8.1.1 Experimental Models of Atrial Arrhythmias

Aconitine induced atrial arrhythmia

Background: Sherf in 1947 used aconitine nitrate to produce arrythmia. He induced atrial fibrillation in dogs by administering (0.05 ml; 0.05 % solution of aconitine nitrate) subpericardially into the area of sinus node. This method induces atrial arrhythmia.

Requirement: Mongrel dogs of either sex (8-12kg), aconite nitrate, chloralose, electro cardiograph (ECG).

Methodology

Dogs are anaesthesized with chloralose (80 mg/kg, i.v). Under artificial respiration through tracheal cannula, heart is exposed by removing part of the sternum and ribs. Pericardial cradle is prepared and cannulation of femoral vein is done for intravenous administration of drugs.

Electro cardiograph is used for recording Lead I, II and III between right and left foreleg, right foreleg and left hind leg, and left foreleg and left hind leg, respectively.

Induction of arrhythmia: Small cotton soaked in 0.05 percent aconitine nitrate is applied to an area, 1-2 mm in diameter on the surface of the atrium. After few minutes persistent atrial fibrillation or flutter is produced.

Administration of drug: Administration of test drug is performed according to the titration procedure that is 1 mg/kg of the drug to be tested is administered intravenously every minute with continuous monitoring of ECG until an arbitrary end point (establishment of 1:1 rhythm with the rate below 200 beats per minute) is achieved.

Note: The test drug is administered after 20 min of the establishment of the atrial arrhythmia.

8.1.2 Experimental Models of Ventricular Arrhythmias

(a) Aconitine induced ventricular arrhythmia in rats

Background: Systemically administered aconitine persistently activates sodium channels. Administered by infusion to anaesthesized rats it can produce ventricular arrhythmias of varying intensity depending on the dose.

Requirements: Wistar/Sprague Dawley rats (180-220 g), 10 animals are used for each dose, aconitine nitrate, urethane, ECG.

Methodology

Anaestheisa: Anaesthetized by i.p. injection of 1.25 g/kg of urethane.

Induction: Aconitine nitrate is dissolved in normal saline and a volume of 5-10 µg/ml is given by slow continuous infusion into the saphenous vein at the rate of 0.1 ml/min.

Recording: Electrocardiogram is recorded every 30 seconds.

Administration: Test drug is intravenously given (3-5 mg/kg). It should be administered 5-10 min before the initiation of aconitine infusion.

Estimation: The anti-arrhythmic activity of a test drug is estimated by the total amount of aconitine used for inducing the following effects:

Extrasystoles of ventricles, ventricular tachycardia, fibrillation of ventricles and death due to ventricular fibrillation

Note: Higher doses of aconitine required for producing these effects in the treated group as compared to controls indicate the anti-arrhythmic potential of test drug.

Evaluation: The results are subjected to statistical test for significance as compared to a standard drug used for comparison.

Note: Aconitine induced atrial and ventricular arrhythmias in dogs and rats respectively are considered valuable screening methods for the evaluation of anti-arrhythmic activity in novel compounds.

(b)   Digoxin-induced ventricular arrhythmias in anesthetized guinea pigs

Background: Higher dose of digoxin produces ventricular extrasystoles, ventricular fibrillation, and finally death. These symptoms may be prevented by anti-arrhythmic drugs.

Requirement: Male guinea pigs (350–450 g), digoxin, pentobarbital, pressure transducer, ECG, lidocaine.

Methodology:

Anesthesia: Pentobarbital sodium (35 mg/kg) is given for anesthesia intraperitoneally.

Cannulation: Cannulation done for jugular vein, trachea and carotid artery.

Artificial respiration: Artificial respiration is given in the form of positive pressure ventilation (45 breaths/ min) using respiratory pump. The carotid artery is used for monitoring systemic blood pressure via a pressure transducer.

Induction of arrhythmia: Arrhythmia is induced by administering digoxin into jugular vein using perfusion pump with the rate of 85 µg/kg in 0.266 ml/min until cardiac arrest.

ECG recording: The ECG recording is done through electro-cardiograph (lead III) with subcutaneous steel-needle electrodes.

Administration of drug: Before digoxin infusion, test drug is given 1 h prior if administered orally and test drug is given 1 min prior if administered intravenously. Standard drugs are lidocaine (3 mg/kg, i.v.) or ramipril (1 mg/kg, p.o).

Recording: The recording is done for ventricular fibrillation, ventricular extrasystoles and cardiac arrest.

Calculation: The total amount of infused digoxin (mg/kg) to induce ventricular fibrillation is calculated.

Evaluation: The doses of digoxin needed to induce ventricular extrasystoles, or ventricular fibrillation, or cardiac arrest, after treatment with anti-arrhythmic drugs are compared statistically with controls receiving digoxin only.

8.1.3 Mechanically Induced Arrhythmias

Mechanical activity in the ischemic region causes membrane depolarization that induces spontaneous arrhythmia. Coronary artery occlusion and ligation induces the ventricular arrhythmia. Reperfusion arrhythmia and coronary occlusion method are some models for mechanical induced Arrythmia.

8.1.4 Chemically Induced Arrhythmias

Involves different types of arrhythmogenic agents. They include anaesthetic like ether, chloroform, halothane and others like adrenaline, acetylcholine, aconitine, cardiac glycosides or veratrum alkaloids.

(a) **Strophanthin K or ouabain induced arrhythmia**

Background: Over dose of strophanthin K or ouabain produces ventricular tachycardia and multifocal ventricular arrhythmias in dogs. This model is used to screen antiarrythmic drugs.

Requirements: Male or female dogs (20 kg), strophanthin K, pentobarbital sodium.

Anesthesia: Pentobarbital sodium (30-40 mg/kg) is given for anesthesia intravenously.

Methodology: Inducing agent and test drugs are given by cannulation of two peripheral veins, individually.

Induction of arrhythmia: Arrhrythmia is induced by administering Stropanthin K by continuous intravenous infusion at a rate of 3 µg/kg/min.

Termination of infusion: The sign of cardiac toxicity in the form of ventricular tachycardia or ventricular arrhythmias is the point of termination of strophanthin infusion.

Administration of drug: Test substance is given in the two different doses of 1.0 and 5.0 mg/kg intravenously when the arrhythmias are stable for 10 min.

ECG recording: ECG recordings are performed at 0.5, 1, 2, 5 and 10 min after administration of test drug.

Efficacy of test drug: Disappearance of extra-systoles is the indication of anti-arrhythmic effect of test compound.

Note: Quinidine, lidocaine and ajmaline are the standard drugs given in the dose of 3 and 10 mg/kg intravenously for re-establishment of normal sinus rhythm.

(b) Adrenaline induced arrhythmia

Background: High dose of adrenaline produces arrhythmia. This model is used to screen anti-arrhythmic drugs.

Requirements: Dogs (10-11 kg, either sex), adrenaline, pento-barbitone sodium.

Methodology: Animals are anaesthetized with pentobarbitone sodium at a dose of 30-40 mg/kg i.p. Femoral vein of the animal is cannulated. Adrenaline is administered 3 min prior to test drug. Adrenaline is administered at a dose of (2-2.5 mg/kg) through the femoral vein. Lead II ECG and atrial ECG are also recorded.

Efficacy of test drug: Test compound is considered to have an anti-arrhythmic effect if the extra-systoles immediately vanished.

8.1.5 Electrically Induced Arrhythmia

Ventricular fibrillation electrical threshold

Background: Electric stimulation leads to fibrillation. Some anti arrhythmic dugs can be screened with this model.

Requirement: Dogs of either sex (10-11 kg), pentobarbitone sodium (30-40 mg/kg, i.p.)

Methodology: Animals are anaesthetized with pentobarbitone sodium at a dose of 30-40 mg/kg; i.p. Animals are provided with an artificial respiration. Blood pressure and temperature are monitored. Chest opened and heart is suspended in pericardial cradle. The SA node is crushed and Ag-Agcl electrode is implanted in Teflon disc. This is joined to arterial surface of left ventrical. The current (3 m sq) is provided through the electrode (400 ms). Digital stimulator is used to program the electrical stimulation. A recording electrode is placed on surface of each ventricle. To determine ventricular fibrillation threshold, 0.2-1.8 train of 50 Hz pulses are delivered 100ms after every 18th stimulus. This induces ventricular fibrillation and drug is administered through femoral vein after 15-20 min recovery time. Ventricular fibrillation is compared before and after drug administration.

8.2 Antihypertensive Activity

Hypertension is the cardiovascular disease. Hypertension is of two types primary and secondary. Arterial hypertension causes damage of blood vessels in heart, kidney and brain. It leads to an increased occurrence of coronary failure, renal failure, and stroke. The screening model for hypertension depends upon kidney, dietary intake of salt and sucrose and there are some genetic models. Figure 8.1 depicts about Renin angiotensin cascade.

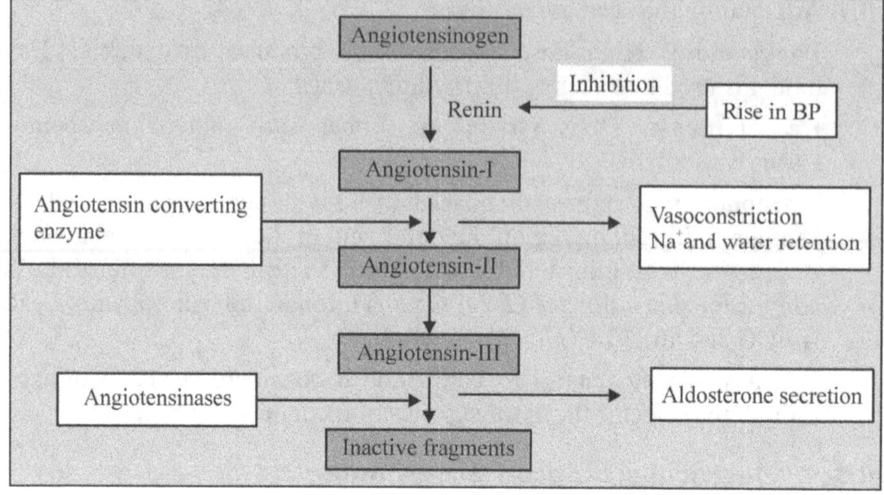

Figure 8.1 Renin angiotensin system.

8.2.1 Experimental Models to Induce Hypertension

(a) Acute renal hypertension in rats (Two –kidney-one-clip)

Background: Goldblatt (1934) has developed two kidney one clip method. Clamped renal artery for 4 hr induces acute renal hypertension. This model is used to screen antihypertensive drugs.

Requirements: Sprague Dawley rats (150-220 g), hexobarbital sodium (100 mg/kg), PVC coated clip.

Methodology: Sprague Dawley rats are anaesthetized with phenobarbitone sodium (50 mg/kg; i.p.). Renal artery is occluded for 4 h by placing a PVC coated clip into left hilum of the kidney and fixed into back muscles. Cannulation of trachea and jugular vein are performed to facilitate spontaneous respiration and administration of test compound, respectively. Renal arterial clip is removed which leads to rise in blood pressure due to elevated plasma renin level [Figure. 8.1]. The test compound is administered by i.v route at a dose of 10 and 100 mg/kg. For each dose of test drug minimum 10 rats are used. Percentage inhibition of the increased blood pressure due to test drug administration is calculated in comparison to pre-treatment hypertension values.

(b) Chronic renal hypertension in rats (one-kidney-one-clip method)

Background: 1-kidney-1-clip model is a modification of Goldblatt et al. (1934). Ischemia of the kidneys induces hypertension. This model is used to induce chronic hypertension.

Requirements: Sprague Dawley rats (180-220g), pentobarbital, U-shaped silver clip.

Methodology: Sprague Dawley rats are anaesthetized with pentobarbital (50 mg/kg, i.p).The fur on the back is shaved and incision is made on the back. The renal pedicel is uncovered with the kidney retracted to the abdomen. The renal artery is dissected and a U-shaped silver clip is fixed around it near the aorta. The right kidney is detached via a flank incision after that renal pedicle is tied off. The skin incision is closed by wound clips. 4-5 weeks after clipping blood pressure is measured. Those rats are selected which have blood pressure higher than 150 mm of Hg. Drugs are administered orally for 3 days. Blood pressure is measured pre-drug and 2 hr post-drug treatment.

Evaluation: Efficacy of the test drug is determined by comparing treatment blood pressure values with the control blood pressure value.

(c)   DOCA salt induced hypertension in rats

Background: Mineralocorticoids administration can lead to hypertension due to their sodium retention property which in turn increases plasma and extracellular volume. This hypertensive effect can be further enhanced by simultaneous salt loading and unilateral nephrectomy in rats.

Requirements: Sprague Dawley rats (180-220g), ether, desoxy-corticosterone acetate (DOCA), olive oil.

Methodology

Sprague Dawley rats are anaesthetized by ether and left kidney is removed through a flank incision.

Induction of hypertension: These unilaterally nephrectomised rats are then treated with 20 mg/kg desoxycorticosterone acetate in olive oil, subcutaneously twice weekly for 4 weeks.

Drinking water is replaced with a 1% sodium chloride solution.

Recording: Blood pressure of these animals start rising towards the end of first week of treatment and the systolic blood pressure reaches 160-180 mm Hg after four weeks.

Evaluation: These hypertensive rats can be then used for the evaluation of antihypertensive activity of test drugs.

(d)   Fructose induced hypertension in rats

Background: Excessive intake of glucose or sucrose in the diet can produce a rise in blood pressure in experimental animals.

Requirements: Male Wistar rats (180-250g), 10% fructose solution

Methodology

Animals are subjected to 12 h light and 12 h dark cycle and are allowed free access to standard rat chow diet and the drinking fluid consisting of either tap water or a 10% fructose solution. Animals are observed daily for body weight, food intake and fluid intake during the treatment.

Sampling: Blood samples are taken before starting the treatment and every second week thereafter and plasma levels of glucose, insulin and trigylcerides are monitored.

Measurement: Using tail cuff method, systolic blood pressure and pulse rate are also recorded simultaneously. Maximum effect on blood pressure and other parameters are achieved after 6 weeks of this treatment.

Evaluation: The hypertensive rats are then used for screening the antihypertensive activity of test drugs.

8.3   Antianginal Drugs

Introduction

Angina pectoris is severe chest pain syndrome that occurs due to the imbalance between oxygen demand of the heart and the oxygen requirement via the coronary blood vessels. The organic nitrates like nitroglycerine is the main drug therapy for the instantaneous relief of angina. For the prophylaxis, calcium channel blockers (vasodilators) and β - blockers are used in the treatment of angina pectoris.

The imbalance between oxygen delivery and utilization may be due to the spasm of the vascular smooth muscle or from obstruction of blood vessels caused by atherosclerotic lesions. Angina is characterized by a sudden, severe pressing substernal pain radiating to the left arm. Three forms of angina are recognized:

(a) **Classical angina (stable angina):** It is a common form of angina, attacks are predictably provoked by exercise, emotion, eating or coitus and settle when the oxygen demand is decreased. A primary pathological event involved is arteriosclerotic obstruction of the larger coronary arteries. Drugs that are useful, primarily reduce cardiac work load, they may also cause favorable re-distribution of blood flow to the ischemic areas.

(b) **Unstable angina:** In this form of angina chest pain occur even at rest. A primary reason is similar to classical angina, i.e. arteriosclerotic obstruction. Drug therapy is also similar to the classic angina.

(c) **Variant angina (Prinzmetal's angina):** It is a uncommon form of angina, attacks occur at rest or during sleep and are unpredictable. They are due to recurrent localized coronary vasospasm which may be superimposed on the arteriosclerotic coronary artery disease. Drugs are mainly used for preventing and relieving the coronary vasospasm.

8.3.1 *In Vitro* Models of Angina Pectoris

(a) Isolated heart (Langendorff) technique

Background: The primary principle involved is that heart is perfused in a retrograde direction from the aorta either at constant oxygenated flow or constant pressure. Retrograde perfusion is the most commonly used techniques in the cardiovascular experiments. The longevity of this preparation is one of the main advantage.

Requirements: Guinea pigs (250-400 g), Ringer's solution.

Methodology

Experimental arrangement: Animals are sacrificed by stunning and the heart is removed as quickly as possible and placed in a Ringer's solution at 37°C. Heart tissues are cleaned properly, pericardial and lung tissues associated with heart are removed. A cannula is inserted in to the aorta, tied, placed to a perfusion apparatus and heart is perfused with oxygenated Ringer's solution at a constant pressure of 40 mm of Hg at a temperature of 37°C. A small steel hook with a string is attached to the upper part of the heart.

Administration of drugs: Drugs are injected in to the perfusion medium, after proper washing of the heart tissues.

Observation: Contractile force is measured by a force transducer and recorded on a polygraph, heart rate is measured by chronometer attached with polygraph. The anti anginal effect of the test drug is indicated by an increase in coronary blood flow.

Evaluation: The incidence and duration of ventricular fibrillation, coronary blood flow, ionotropic state and potassium levels after treatment with drug are compared with control.

(b) Calcium antagonism in the isolated rabbit aorta

Background: Addition of potassium chloride or nor-adrenaline to the organ bath containing slightly modified Krebs bicarbonate buffer induces contraction of aorta rings. Test drugs with calcium channel antagonistic activity have a relaxation effect on the rings.

Requirments: Rabbits (3-4kg), Krebs bicarbonate buffer, potassium chloride.

Methodology

Experimental arrangement: Animals are sacrificed with an overdose of pentobarbital sodium. Thoracic aorta is rapidly removed from the chest cavity and placed in the Krebs bicarbonate buffer at 37°C. Eight rings of 4-5 mm width are obtained and each is mounted in 20 ml tissue bath containing Krebs solution. A constant contraction is shown by addition of potassium chloride.

Administration of drugs: Twenty minutes after addition of agonist, the test drug is added. The percent relaxation reading is taken every 30 min after addition of the test drug. There is a 30 min time interval between additions of different test drugs.

Observation: Active tension is calculated for the tissue at time point just prior to the addition of the test compound and also at the point 30 min after the addition of each concentration of the test compound.

Evaluation: Percentage relaxation caused by the test drug from the pre contracted level, is calculated.

(c) Calcium antagonism in pitched rat

Background: Using the cardioacclerator response in pitched rats, calcium channel blockers can be distinguished from other agents, which are not acting directly on the calcium channel.

Requirments: Sprague-Dawley albino rats (150-280 g)

Methodology

Experimental arrangement: Animals are anesthetized with methotrexate sodium (50 mg/kg, i.p). After cannulation of trachea, rats are pitched through one orbit and immediately maintained on artificial respiration.

Administration of drugs: Drugs are administered in the cannulated jugular vein.

Observation: Blood pressure is recorded by carotid artery using a pressure transducer. The cardioacceleration response is obtained by continuous electrical stimulation.

Evaluation: Tachycardial level immediately prior to drug administration is taken as 100% and response to drugs is expressed as percentage of pre-dose tachycardia. ID_{50} is calculated and compared.

(d) Plastic casts from coronary vasculature in dogs

Background: Coronary drug when administered for prolonged duration leads to increase in the number and size of interarterial collaterals, especially in pigs and dogs. Acute or gradual occlusion of one of the major coronary branches may also stimulate development of collaterals.

Requirements: Dogs (10-15 kg), pentobarbital.

Methodology

Experimental arrangement: Animals are anesthetized with pentobarbital sodium (30 mg/kg, i.v) and uphold on the artificial respiration system. After that chest cavity is opened and the heart is exposed, ameroid cuffs are placed around the major coronary branches. A plastic material gradually swells and occludes the lumen within 3 - 4 weeks. After completion of treatment (6 weeks), animals are sacrificed, and their hearts removed and coronary bed flushed with saline.

Observation: Care is taken to maintain the uniformity of the filling pressure and viscosity. After polymerization is complete the tissue is digested with 35% KOH.

Evaluation: Plastic casts from the drug treated animals are compared with casts from the normal group (dogs subjected to the same procedure without drug treatment). The ability of the test drug to increase the number and size of collateral is evaluated.

(e)   Occlusion of coronary artery

Background: Infarct size is studied after proximal occlusion of the coronary artery in open chest dogs. Compounds that reduce infarct size are studied using nitro-blue tetrazolium chloride stain in myocardial sections. Gelatin mass of barium sulphate is injected in to the left coronary, coronary arteriogram are prepared and these studies are used in the area of risk.

Requirments: Dogs of either sex (30 kg), nitro-blue tetrazolium

Methodology

Experimental arrangement: The animals are anesthetized with pentobarbitone sodium (35 mg/kg, i.p), which is followed by continuous infusion at 4 mg/kg/h. Trachea is cannulated and the animal maintained on artificial respiration. Test compound is administered in to the cannulated peripheral vein. ECG is recorded continuously. Cannulated femoral vein is connected to a pressure transducer for measuring peripheral systolic and diastolic pressure. Heart is exposed through left thoractomy between 4th and 5th intercostal space. The pericardium is opened and the left anterior descending coronary artery is exposed and then ligated for 360 min. Test substance or vehicle is administered by intravenous bolus injection.

Observation: Hemodynamic parameters like systolic and diastolic blood pressure are monitored during the protocol, after completion of experimental protocol, animals are sacrificed with an overdose of pentobarbital sodium. Area at risk of infarction is measured using coronary arteriograms. The left ventricle is cut into transverse sections. From each slice angiograms are made with X-ray tube at 40 kv to assess the area at risk of infarction by defect opacity, reduction of $BaSO_4$ filled vessel in infarct tissue. The slices are then incubated in nitro-blue tetrazolium (0.25 g/ l) in order to visualize the area of infarcted tissues.

Evaluation: Normal tissue is blue/violet stained while necrotic tissue appear unstained. Further slices are photographed for determination of infarct area. Mortality, hemodynamic, and size of infarcted area are determined after completion of experiment. These parameters are evaluated in the drug treatment animals and compared to the sham group.

(f) Isoproterenol – induced myocardial necrosis

Background: Synthetic catecholamines, isoproterenol when injected at high dose produce cardiac necrosis. Several drugs such as sympatholytics or calcium channel blockers can totally or partially prevent this necrosis.

Requirments: Wistar albino rats (150-200g), pentobarbital, isoproterenol.

Methodology

Experimental arrangement: Wistar albino rats(150-200g) are pre treated with test drug or standard drug orally for one week. These animals are then injected with isoproterenol (85 mg/kg, s.c) on two successive days. Mortality as well as other parameters are recorded in each group and compared to group injected with isoproterenol only. After 48 h of first dose isoproterenol, the animals are sacrificed. The heart is removed, weighed and preserved for histology and various biochemical parameter evaluation.

Observation: Before sacrificing, the animals hemodynamic parameters like systolic/diastolic blood pressure and heart rate can be recorded by cannulating the carotid artery and connecting it to the pressure transducer.

Evatuation: Changes of hemodynamic histological and biochemical parameters of drug treated animals are compared to the isoproterenol control groups.

(g) Myocardial ischemic preconditioning model

Background: Myocardial ischemic preconditioning can reduce the damage produced by prolonged ischemia and reperfusion. Preliminary preconditioning of the myocardium reduces infarct size, improves post-ischemic ventricular function, as well as attenuates cardiac arrhythmia associated with frequent ischemia/reperfusion.

Requirments: Rabbits (3-4 kg), ketamine.

Methodology

Experimental arrangement: Rabbits are anesthetized with ketamine (50 mg/ml)/xylazine (10 mg/ml) at a dose of 0.6 ml/kg, i.p. Trachea is cannulated and the animal maintained on artificial respiration. The right femoral artery and vein are catheterized for measurement of arterial pressure and administration of drugs respectively. Ischemic preconditioning is induced by tightening the loop around the coronary artery for 5 min and then loosening to reperfuse the myocardium for 10 min prior to the subsequent 30 min occlusion. After 30 min of ischemia, ligature is released for 120 min of reperfusion. Prior to the 30 min of occlusion, the rabbits are selected to receive ischemic preconditioning, no preconditioning or preconditioning along with the administration of the test compound. The animals are sacrificed after the reperfusion duration.

Evaluation: Parameters like systolic, diastolic, mean blood pressure, heart rate left venricular pressure, and left venricular end- diastolic pressure are measured by using ANOVA software.

8.4   Anti-Atherosclerotic Agents

Hyperlipidemia is defined as the presence of high concentration of fats such as cholesterol, cholesterol ester, triglycerides and phospholipids in the blood. Different experimental models for screening anti-atherosclerotic activity are discussed in this section.

(a) Cholesterol- diet induced atherosclerosis

> **Background:** Excessive intake of cholesterol in diet can produce severe hypercholesterolemia and atherosclerosis in rabbits. This classical method has been used for the screening of potential anti-atherosclerotic drugs.

> **Requirements:** New Zealand white rabbits, biochemical analyzer, 2% cholesterol

> **Methodology**

> **Selection of animals:** Male inbred New Zealand white rabbits at the age of 8-10 weeks. 10 animals are used in each group.

> **Isolation of blood:** At the beginning of the experiment blood is withdrawn from the marginal ear vein and baseline values of total serum cholesterol, triglycerides and blood sugar are estimated. First of all rabbits are given normal diet and afterwards replaced with a diet having 2% cholesterol for 10-12 weeks.

> At the end of the test period the blood from all the groups is withdrawn and analyzed.

> **Note:** This method has been modified to produce atherosclerosis in various other animal species like rats, mice, hamster, turkeys and monkeys.

(b) Cholesterol- Diet induced hyperlipidemia in mice

Background: Excessive intake of fat rich diet may lead to hyperlipidemia via increased LDL levels and reduced HDL levels in blood. High cholesterol diet method is well established model to induce hyperlipidemia.

Requirements: Male mice (28-30g), 10% lard, 10% egg yolk powder, 1% cholesterol, 0.2% bile salt, 10%urethane.

Methodology

Experimental arrangement: All mice are provided an identical diet of normal chow during the first week. The mice are given high-fat diet for next 15 days. The food intake is recorded daily and the body weight is recorded every week.

Administration of drug: Test or standard drugs are given to animals with oral gavage, treated daily for 15 days. After 4 weeks treatments, the mice are fasted overnight and anesthetized with 10% urethane (i.p.), the blood samples are collected *via* retro-orbital venous plexus puncture. The collected blood is centrifuged for 2 min at 16000 revolutions per min and serum is isolated for determination of total cholesterol (TC) and triglyceride (TG).

Evaluation: Antihyperlipidemic drugs reduced total cholesterol (TC) and triglyceride (TG). The mean value of serum cholesterol and standard error are calculated for each group and subjected to analysis for statistical significance.

(c) Triton induced hyperlipidemia

Background: Triton administration to rats and mice leads to biphasic elevation of plasma cholesterol and triglycerides. Triton increases cholesterol synthesis in liver. Triton inhibits the uptake of plasma lipids by other tissues of the body.

Requirements: Male Wistar rats (150-220g), Triton WR 1339 (iso-octyl-polyoxyethylenephenol),

Methodology

Experimental arrangement: Animals are starved for 18 h prior to administration of Triton WR 1339 (iso-octyl-polyoxyethylenephenol).

Phase-I response: Triton at a dose of 200mg/kg raises the level of serum cholesterol after 24 h of administration

Phase-II response: The hypercholesterolemia reduces to normal within the next 24 h. The test drugs are injected along with Triton.

Evaluation: Mean values of serum cholesterol and standard error are calculated for each group and subjected to analysis for statistical significance.

(d) Fructose induced hypertriglyceridemia in rats

Background: Fructose (20%) orally daily given to rats leads to induction of significant hypertriglyceridemia which can be used for screening of antihyperlipedemic compounds.

Requirements: Protein rich diet, 20% fructose solution, anesthetic ether

Methodology:

Selection of animals: Male Wistar rats or Sprague Dawley rats (180-220g)

Administration of drug: First of all rats are maintained on a diet with less carbohydrates and high proteins and then they are given high amount of fructose. Test or standard drugs are given to animals with oral gavage, treated daily for 3 days. On 2nd and 3rd day water is withheld too. Immediately animals are offered 20% fructose solution *ad libitium* for a period of 24 h.

Isolation of blood: After 20 h of last test compound administration, the animals are anaesthetized with ether and 1.2 ml of blood is withdrawn by retro-orbital puncture. The collected blood is centrifuged for 2 min at 16000 revolutions per min.

Evaluation: Total glycerol and total cholesterol are estimated in the serum and compared for statistical significance.

8.5   Antiplatelet Activity

Blood vessels get occluded due to deposition of platelets on surfaces of thrombogens. This condition is related to several pathological modifications in the body i.e. unstable angina, acute myocardial infarction, stroke and ischemic complication of coronary intervention. Platelet aggregation occur due to arterial wall injury. The agonists activate platelets for their adherence and aggregation to injured blood vessels surface that leads to formation of occlusive thrombus in the lumen of the vessel. Aggregation of platelets occurs due to stimulation of thrombin, collagen, serotonin, thromboxane A2 and combination of all these factors. The agents used for inducing aggregation of platelets for drug screening models are discussed below.

(a) Photochemically induced thrombosis model in rats

Background: Photochemical reaction can induce thrombosis. This is very useful screening model for anti thrombotic agents.

Requirments: Albino Wistar rat (either sex, 150-220 g), sodium pentobarbital, surgical kit.

Methodology: Male albino rats (150-220 g) are anesthetized with sodium pentobarbital (60 mg/kg, i.p) injected into the femoral muscle.

The right jugular vein and artery are cannulated for the injection of dye and the monitoring of arterial blood pressure and heart rate, respectively. Thrombus formation is induced in micro vessels by a filtered light of wavelength 420-490 nm passed through an object.

The test agent is administered by i.v. bolus injection in to the jugular vein of the rat. One minute after the injection irradiation with filtered light is started. One minute after the start of irradiation, a solution of sodium fluorescein (2.5% w/v) is injected through the jugular vein (1 ml/kg body weight). Whole process is monitored with TV camera after injection of sodium fluorescein. The time when the thrombus begins to form and the time when blood flow completely stops are used as indices of antithrombotic activity. Time is measured by replay of the videotape. If the blood flow does not stop within 30 min, the result is calculated as 30 min.

8.6   Cardiotonic Drugs Activity

Cardiotonic drugs increase the contraction of heart muscle. It increases blood flow to all the tissues. It basically has a positive ionotropic effect. Increased force of contraction increases the amount of blood leaving the left ventricle at each contraction cycle and thus increases the cardiac output. These drugs are used for congestive heart failure (CHF), myocardial infarction, and cardiac surgical procedure. Failure of heart can be identified by the reduction in ejection fraction and dysfunction of diastoles. Infarction in heart occurs due to reduced blood flow that causes damage to the muscles of heart. Cardiotonics may be a cardiac glycosides or cardiac stimulants.

Cardiac glycosides: Digitalis

Cardiac stimulant

(a) Sympathomimetic agents: adrenaline, dobutamine, dopamine

(b) Phosphodiesterase inhibitors: amrinone, milrinone

8.6.1 *In Vitro* Method

(a) **Isolated hamster cardiomyopathic heart**

Background: Isolated heart of Syrian hamster is used to evaluate the cardiotonic drugs.

Requirement: Hamster (50 week old), ringer's solution

Methodology: Hamster with cardiomyopathy is used as test group. Normal Syrian hamsters (50 week old) are used as control. Animals are treated with heparin and after 20 minutes the heart is prepared according to the method of Langendorff. Later the heart is perfused with Ringer's solution. Further it is equilibrated for 60 min with a load of 1.5 grams in the isolated state. Force of contraction is recorded by a force transducer. The heart rate is measured using an instrument chronometer. The coronary flow is measured with the help of electro-flow meter. Test compounds are administered into the Ringer solution with the help of aortic cannula.

8.6.2 *In Vivo* Models

(a) Rat coronary ligation model

Background: Left coronary artery is ligated which results in heart failure may be due to chronic myocardial ischaemia.

Requirement: Sprague Dawley rats (150-220g), hexobarbital

Methodology: Male Sprague Dawley rats are anaesthetised with hexobarbital (200 mg/kg). Trachea is cannulated and animal is given artificial respiration. Chest cavity is exposed and the left anterior descending (LAD) carotid artery is isolated. Ligature is placed around the LAD and the chest cavity is sutured back and animal maintained on food and water. After 4 weeks chest cavity is opened and carotid artery as well as jugular vein is cannulated for measurement of blood pressure as well as administration of test compound. Systolic, diastolic and mean blood pressure is measured. After measuring the hemodynamic parameter the animals are sacrificed and the isolated hearts are used for estimation of calcium and calcium ATPase level.

(b) Spontaneously hypertensive heart failure rats (SH-HF)

Background: Breeding is done for spontaneously hypertensive rats that develop failure of heart prior to achieve 18 months of age due to the gene presence of gene facp. This gene encodes defective leptin receptor (SH-HF/Mcc-facp). The activities shown by this rat are increased atrial natriuretic peptide, aldosterone level and renin plasma activity.

Requirements: Spontaneously hypertensive rats

Methodology: Animals are grouped into test group and control group. In the test group drug is administered orally for one month. After completion of the experiment both the groups are compared for their plasma renin activity, AMP and aldosterone level.

(c) Dahl salt sensitive rats

Background: This strain of rat develops systemic hypertension after receiving a high salt diet.

Requirements: Dahl salt sensitive rats (150-240 g), 1% NaCl solution.

Methodology

Dahl salt sensitive rats are provided 1% NaCl solution in place of drinking water. Rats are given food which is prepared by mixing salt with regular diet. Rats are provided dahl salt diet and 1% NaCl solution. Animals are grouped into test and sham control groups. Test compound is administered orally for 1 month. After completion of protocol, animals of both the groups are sacrificed. Hearts of these animals are removed and total cardiac mass and weights of left and right ventricles are recorded.

8.6.3 Rabbit Models of Heart Failure

Rabbit model is used for the heart failure has many similarity with the human heart.

(a) Volume and pressure overload

Background: Volume and pressure overload are used to induce heart failure in rabbits.

Requirements: Rabbit (1.5- 3kg), pentobarbitone sodium

Methodology: Animals are anesthetized with pentobarbitone sodium (35 mg/kg, i.p.). Trachea is cannulated and animals are maintained on artificial respiration. Carotid artery is cannulated. Chest cavity is opened and heart is exposed. Aortic insufficiency is produced by destroying aortic valves with the catheter. Chest cavity is sutured back. Animals are administered antibiotic to stop any kind of infection. After 2 weeks, below the diaphragm aorta is constricted with a clamp. Test drugs are administered for 14 days. After 4 weeks heart failure occurs which is confirmed by checking the aortic constriction. After completion of the experiment, various parameters are measured such as protein, mRNA levels of the Na^+Ca^{2+} exchanger and compared in test groups and control groups.

8.6.4 Guinea Pig Model

(a) Aortic banding

Background: CHF in guinea pigs are induced by banding the descending thoracic aorta. It mimics heart failure similar to human.

Requirements: Male guinea pigs (300-450 g), ether, rubber tube

Methodology: Guinea pigs are anaesthetized with ether. Chest cavity is opened, pericardium is removed and heart is exposed. Extrusion of beating heart is done from the thorax. To keep the heart outside the thorax, it is placed on a base covered with a thin rubber tube and clamped with ring, so that it does not interfere with the blood circulation. To tie the apical third of both ventricles of heart, a thread is used that is previously soaked in a disinfectant. Again the heart is placed back and clamp is removed. Incision is performed between the 4th and 5th costal ribs. Air is removed from the thorax. Test drug is administered for two weeks. The animals develop symptoms of CHF with death rate of 80% within one day. Heart weight and lung weight are compared for both the groups. Lung edema and liver congestion are observed histologically.

8.6.5 Syrian Hamster Model

(a) Cardiomyopathic hamster

Background: Syrian hamsters are widely used for heart failure and cardiac hypertrophy. An autosomal recessive mode of inheritance is exhibited by this model that leads to degenerative lesion in all striated muscle, particularly in the myocardium.

Requirements: Syrian hamster (50-80g).

Methodology: Syrian hamsters develop heart failure after 7-10 months. Necrotic and calcified myocardial lesions are observed during the initial development of disease. Cardiomyopathic disease is characterized by little fibrosis, calcium deposition, hypertrophy of the myocyte and a final stage of depressed myocardial performance and failure. Test drugs are administered to the animals for a period of 14 days through the preferred route. Test drugs are evaluated on the basis of above mentioned characteristic feature. Benefit of this model is that no surgery is needed for the evaluation.

8.6.6 Dog Models of Heart Failure

(a) Chronic rapid pacing

Background: In healthy dogs heart rate is increased above 200 beats/min for within several weeks produces the syndrome of heart failure.

Requirements: Male dogs (18 to 25 kg), pentobarbital.

Methodology: Adult male dogs are anaesthetized with pentobarbital (30 mg/kg, i.p.). Animals are maintained on artificial respiration. Chest cavity is opened and the heart is exposed (through thoracotomy). A ventricular lead is joined to the left ventricular apex. Pacemaker is also attached at a pace of 240 to 260 beats/min. Heart is placed back in the chest cavity after the surgical procedure. Air is removed from the thorax. Antibiotic emulsion is applied on the wound. Heart failure start to develop after 4 weeks and persist up to 10 weeks. Comparison between test group and sham control group is made on the basis of changes in parameters like ejection fraction, cardiac output.

(b) Volume overload

Background: Prolonged volume overload may lead to development of heart failure.

Requirements: Dogs (15-20 kg), Pentobarbital

Methodology: Dogs are anesthetized with pentobarbital (30 mg/kg; i.p.). Animals are maintained on artificial respiration. Thoracotomy is performed and the heart is exposed. After the surgical procedure, heart is placed back in the chest cavity and the costal ribs closed. Air in the thoracic cavity is removed. Antibiotic emulsion is applied on the wound. Heart failure develops after 4 weeks and continues for up to 10 weeks. Test drugs are administered for a period of 14 days. After completion of experiment comparison between test animals and control animals is made. Dogs with CHF myocardial function is depressed and renin angiotensin system activation occurs. These characteristic features are compared in both the groups.

References

- Rees, D. A., Alcolado, J.C. Animal models of diabetes mellitus.Diabet Med.2004; 22 (4) : 359-370.

- Sharma, R., et. al. Experimental models on diabetes: A comprehensive review.IJAPS. 2013; 4 (1) : 01-08.

- Gupta, S. K., 2004. Drug screening methods. Jaypee brothers medical publishers LTD. New Delhi; pp. 195-206, 208-214, 236-246.

- Srinivasan K, Ramarao P. Animal models in type 2 diabetes research: An overview. IJMR. 2007; 125(3):451-472.

- Etuk, E. U. Animals models for studying diabetes mellitus.ABJNA. 2007; 125 (3) : 451-472.

- Vogel, G. H., 2002. Drug Discovery and evaluation: Pharmacological assays. Springer-verlag berlin Heidelberg publication. New York; pp. 209-227.

Chapter 9

Evaluation of Drugs Acting on Endocrine System

9.1 Anti Diabetic Activity

Diabetes mellitus (DM) is a metabolic disorder which is characterized by hyperglycemia, hyperlipidemia and glycosuria. Symptoms of diabetes mellitus may be frequent urination, increased thirst and increased hunger.

- **Type 1 DM:** In this type of diabetes mellitus there is 90% destruction of β cells and there is less production of insulin. Type 1 of DM is also known as the "Insulin-Dependent Diabetes Mellitus" (IDDM) or "Juvenile Diabetes".

- **Type 2 DM:** Type 2 DM mainly results from insulin resistance. In this situation body is producing enough insulin but it cannot utilize it. Type 2 DM is also known as "Non-Insulin-Dependent Diabetes Mellitus" (NIDDM) or "Adult-onset Diabetes".

Gestational diabetes – It occurs mainly in pregnant women, with no history of diabetes. After parturition the blood glucose level becomes normal. It is very troublesome. Diabetes may recur in later period of life.

9.1.1 Methods to Induce Experimental Diabetes Mellitus

(a) Streptozotocin induced diabetes

Streptozotocin [2-Deoxy-2-(3-methyl-3-nitrosoureido)-D-glucopyranose] (STZ) is a broad spectrum antibiotic isolated from *Streptomyces achromogenes* in 1959. STZ enters the pancreatic cell via a glucose transporter-GLUT2 and causes alkylation of DNA. Chemical structure of Streptozotocin is depicted in Figure 9.1.

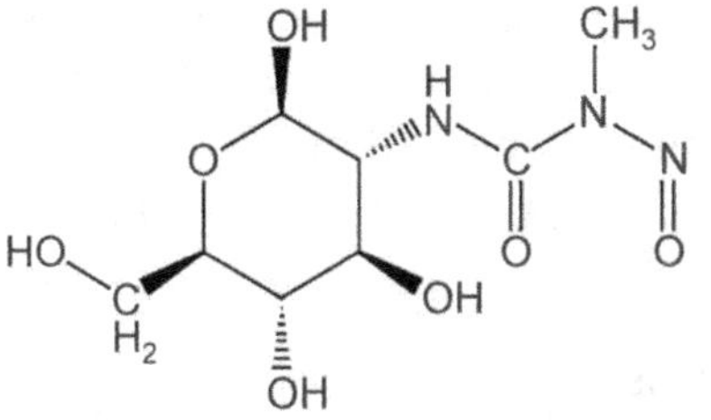

Figure 9.1 Structure of streptozotocin.

Background: STZ induces diabetes in almost all the species because it has cytotoxic action to pancreatic β cells. In most species triphasic response is observed.

- Initially the blood glucose level increases to 150-200 mg/dL within 3 hr.

- A phase of hypoglycemia occurs due to four-fold increase in serum insulin levels in 6-8 hours.

- This phase is later followed by persistent hyperglycemia.

- **Requirement:** Albino rats (160-180 g), streptozotocin, chow diet, water

Methodology:

- **Administration of test drug:** Streptozotocin (60 mg/kg, i.p.) is administered to these rats by intraperitoneal injection.

- **Induction of diabetes:** Whether diabetes has been induced or not is confirmed by checking the blood glucose level with Glucometer after 3 days or by UV methods. If the blood glucose level is above 220 mg/dl then the animal is considered diabetic. A steady state hyperglycemia reaches after 10-14 days when these animals can be used for the pharmacological screening of test compound.

(b) Alloxan induced diabetes

Background: Alloxan is chemically known as 5, 5-dihydroxyl pyrimidine-2,4,6-trione. It induces hyperglycemia in various species including dogs, rats and rabbits. It also produces triphasic response like streptozotocin. Alloxan produces diabetes via its cytotoxic action on pancreatic β cells due to accumulation of reactive oxygen species. These reactive oxygen species further gets converted into hydrogen peroxide which leads to formation of reactive hydroxyl radical and causes destruction of β cells.

Requirement: Healthy rabbits (2.0 to 3.5 kg) and / or Albino rats (150-200g), Alloxan monohydrate.

Methodology

Administration of drug: In rabbits, alloxan monohydrate (150 mg/kg) is infused via ear vein. In rats, alloxan is given at a dose of (100-200 mg/kg, s.c). In dogs alloxan at the dose of (60 mg/kg, i.v) induces diabetes. Alloxan is administered at different doses sometimes single dose and sometimes at graded doses (2-3 dose).

Disadvantages of chemically induced diabetes

- Chemicals are toxic to other parts of the body.

- Mortality rate is high.

- Blood glucose level may become normal after few weeks.

(c) Genetically diabetic animals

Background: Due to mutation in insulin 2 gene, diabetes is induced in some rats and mice. They are known as genetically diabetic animals. Mutation in insulin 2 gene stops the correct processing of pro insulin. Due to this there is an excess misfolded protein which leads to subsequent ER stress. Diabetes is induced from 3 to 4 weeks of age. It is characterized by hyperglycemia, hypoinsulinemia, polyuria and polydipsia. Untreated animals cannot survive after 12 weeks of age, example of genetically diabetic animal is Akita mouse. Akita mouse is derived from Akita, Japan. Non obese diabetic mouse (NOD): NOD mouse is derived in Japan, which is an inbred strain.

(d) Spontaneous diabetic rats

Background: Spontaneous diabetic rats signifies such type of diabetic rats in which diabetes is genetically transferred from one generation to another generation such as bio breeding rats and Cohen diabetic rats.

Bio breeding rats (BB): BB rats is derived from outbred rats. In BB rat model diabetes is inherited with recessive trait. The onset of diabetes is sudden, and occurs at about 60-120 days of age. The diabetic animals get severe hyperglycemia, hypoinsulinemia and ketonic condition unless insulin treatment is instituted.

Cohen diabetic rat: In Cohen diabetic rat's glucosurea, hyperinsulinemia, and hyperglycemia are the most important features.

(e) Surgically induced diabetes

Background: Diabetes is induced by surgical removal of all parts of the pancreas. Removal of pancreas leads to destruction of α, β, and δ cells. Removal of all parts of pancreas leads to insulin dependent diabetes mellitus. Depending on remaining intact pancreatic tissue, blood glucose level may become normal or remains high for longer duration.

9.2   Antifertility Activity

The combined oral contraceptives (COCs) were first launched in market in 1961. Progestins alone pills are effective contraceptives as they inhibit gonadotropin secretion, suppress the mid cycle LH surge and stops ovulation. They also induce atrophy of endometrial glands, thickening of cervical mucus and decrease the tubal motility and thus reduce fertility. In spite of the COCs being successfully used for decades, there is the need for a long acting and safe oral contraceptive agents, which may suit the convenience of women and offer greater compliance. Estrus cycle and way to hold a female rat to take out smear is shown in Figure 9.2 and 9.3 respectively.

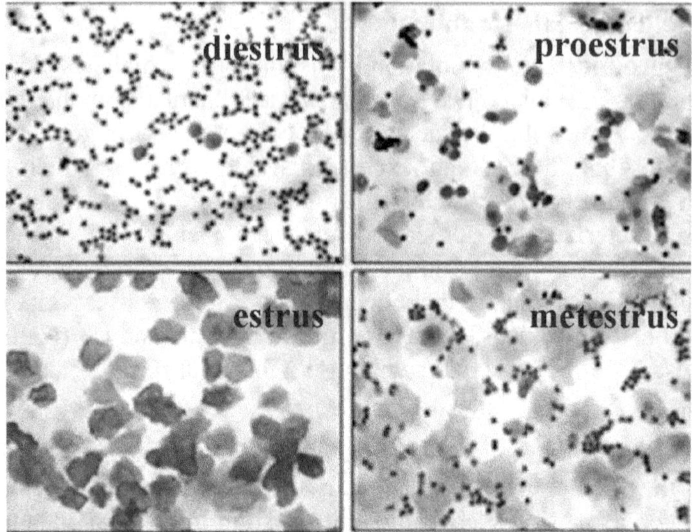

Figure 9.2 Estrus cycle.

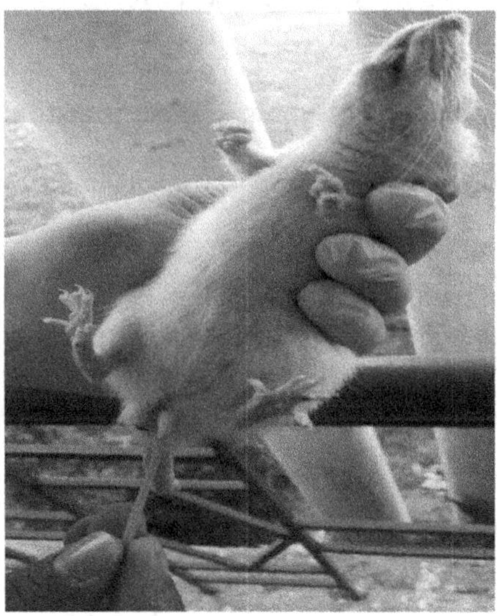

Figure 9.3 Way to hold the female rat to examine smear

9.2.1 Female Rat Estrus Cycle

Estrus cycle last for four days. It is divided into four phases. Metestrus, diestrus, proestrus and estrus. Because of small estrus cycle, changes occurring during the reproductive cycle are examined easily. These phases of the cycle are distinguished by cell present in the smear.

Metestrus: Smear consist of same proportion of cornified, leukocyte and nucleated epithelial cells. Ovarian hormone secretion is relatively low and follicular activity starts. Metestrus cycle last for 21 h.

Diestrus: Smear consist of a predominance of leukocytes. Follicle continues to develop and there is a significant increase in estrogen level. Diestrus cycle last for 57 h.

Proestrus: Smear consist of predominance of nucleated epithelial cells. Estradiol level is maximum. Proestrus cycle last for about 12h.

Estrus: Smear consist of anucleated cornified cells. Prolactin, LH and FSH level remains low. Estrus cycle last for about 12 h.

9.2.2 Models to Screen Anti-Fertility Drugs

(a) Inhibition of ovulation in rats

Background: This method has been used for the assay of progestrogens steroids. Progesterone receptors (PR) are activated by these steroid hormones. Progesterone (P4) is the important progestrogen in the body. Repeated administration of progestogens inhibits ovulation and corpus lutea formation in young female rats by decreasing the secretion of LH.

Requirements: Albino female rats (35 -40 days old), progesterone, dissection instruments

Methodology:

Animals are treated daily with (0.5 to 2.0 mg of progesterone; s/c). On 8th day, the animals are sacrificed and body weight, ovary weight and number of corpus luteum are recorded.

Progestogens reduces ovarian weight and inhibit corpus luteum formation. Corpus luteum is an endocrine structure. Corpus luteum maintains the uterus. The number of corpus luteum is directly proportional to oogenesis.

(b) Antagonism of uterus weight

Background: Increase of uterine weight in castrated female rats induced by estradiol can be antagonized by antiestrogenic compounds.

Requirements: Female rats, estradiol,

Methodolgy: Female rats are ovariectomised. Control rats are injected with estradiol 0.03-0.06 µg/animals for 7 days. The test compounds are also administered in various groups for 7 days. On 8th day, animals are sacrificed. Uterus is removed and weight of the uterus is noted down. The antiestrogenic effect is expressed as:

Percent (%) reduction of estrogen = Stimulated uterine weight by the test compounds compared to rats treated with estradiol alone.

(c) Antiimplantation activity in the female rats

Background: Anti-implantation effects can be demonstrated in female rats by treating them with test drug and comparing with control group.

Requirements: Sprague-Dawley or Wistar rats (150-200 g), anesthetic agents, test drug.

Methodology: Female rats in proestrus phase are kept with male rats of proven fertility in the ratio of 2:1. The female rats are examined in the following morning for presence of spermatozoa in vaginal smear. The detection of spermatozoa in vaginal smear is considered as day 1 of pregnancy. The pregnant animals are divided into four groups (n=6). Animals in the groups I is given vehicle only and serve as control. The test drug is administered at three different doses to group II, III and group IV respectively from day 1 to 7 of pregnancy. On 8th day all the animals are sacrificed under light anesthesia and laprotomy is performed to determine the number of implantation sites on the both uterine horns and the number of corpora lutea (represents number of eggs ovulated) on both ovaries. The antiimplantation activity is calculated by the percentage of implantation per number of corpora leutea.

(d) Antifertility activity in female rats

Background: Antifertility effects can be demonstrated in female rats by treating them with test drug and comparing with control group.

Requirements: Female Sprague-Dawley or Wistar rats (150-200 g), anesthetic agents, test drug.

Methodology: The pregnant rats are selected (as discussed under antiimplantation activity) and are divided into the four groups, a control group and three experimental groups (n=6). On 10th day of pregnancy animals are laprotomised under light anesthesia using sterile condition. Both the horns of uteri are observed to determine the implantation sites. The abdominal wound is sutured using catgut. Post operational care is taken to avoid any infection. The test drug is given at three different doses orally from day 11 to day 15 of pregnancy. The animals are allowed to go full term. After delivery the litters are counted and the antifertility activity is calculated. Pups are also examined for any malformations.

References

- Rees, D. A., Alcolado, J.C. Animal models of diabetes mellitus. Diabet Med. 2004; 22 (4): 359-370.
- Sharma, R., et. al. Experimental models on diabetes: A comprehensive review. IJAPS. 2013; 4 (1): 01-08.

- Srinivasan K, Ramarao P. Animal models in type 2 diabetes research: An overview. IJMR. 2007; 125 (3): 451-472.

- Etuk, E. U. Animals models for studying diabetes mellitus. ABJNA. 2007; 125 (3): 451-472.

- Vogel, G. H., 2002. Drug Discovery and evaluation: Pharmacological assays. Springer-verlag berlin Heidelberg publication. New York; pp. 209-227, 85-104.

- Gupta, S. K., 2004. Drug screening methods. Jaypee brothers medical publishers LTD. New Delhi; pp. 236-246.

- Johns, C., Gavras, I. Models of experimental hypertension in mice. Hypertension. 1996; 28 (6): 1064-1069.

- Badyal, D. K., Lata, H., Dadhich, A. P. Animal Models of hypertension and effect of drugs. Indian J Pharmacol. 2003; 35 (6): 349-362.

- Goldstein, J. L., Brown, M. S. The LDL receptor locus and the genetics of familiar hypercholesterolemia. Annu. Rev. Genet.1979; 13:258-289.

- Brown, M. S., Goldstein, J. L. Familial hypercholesterolemia: Model for genetic receptor disease. Med Clin N Amer.1979; 73:163-20.

- Marcondes, F. K., Bianchi, F. J. Tanno, A. P. Determination of the estrus cycle phases of rats: some helpful considerations. Braz. J. Biol. 2002; 62(4): 609-614.

- Shivayogi H.P., Shrishailappa B., Swamy H.K.S., Saraswati P.B and Ramesh L. L. Antifertility Activity of *Striga orobanchioides*. Biol.Pharm. Bull. 1994; 17(8): 1029-31.

Chapter 10

Evaluation of Drug Acting on Kidney

10.0 Kidney

Kidney regulates the excretion of solutes and water. It also regulates the homeostasis. It indirectly regulates blood pressure and renin angiotensin system. It secretes a variety of hormones. There are various animal models which gives us the information about acute renal failure (ARF). Acute renal failure (ARF) is basically less renal functioning, fall in glomerular filtration rate (GFR) and slow excretion of nitrogenous waste.

10.1 Experimental Models for Diuretic and Saluretic Activity

(a) Patch clamp technique in kidney cells (*in vitro* method)

Background: The principle behind this model is that fluid gets reabsorbed from the different parts of the kidney and substances may be transported either from the tubule lumen to the blood side (reabsorption) or vice versa (secretion). Ion channels play an important role in the urine formation.

Requirements: Rabbit kidney cells, patch pipette, patch electrode, gigaseals, glass pipette, collagenase, HEPES, calcium chloride, magnesium chloride, homogenizer

Methodology

Cell culture:

The method of patch clamping is used for cultured kidney cells or freshly isolated kidney cells. The segments of proximal tubules of rabbit kidney are dissected and perfused with a perfusion system from one end. A patch pipette makes the noncannulated end of the tubule freely accessible. Under optical control the patch pipette can be moved through the open end into the tubule lumen and is brought in contact with the brush border membrane. After slight suction of the patch electrode, gigaseals form instantaneously and single potassium or sodium channels can be recorded in the cell-attached or inside-out cell-excised mode. Pieces of the tubule are torn off by means of a glass pipette (diameter about 40 μm) the tubules are incubated for about 5 min in 0.5 g/l collagenase at room temperature. After tearing off part of the cannulated tubule, clean lateral cell membranes are exposed at the non-cannulated end. After cervical dislocation the kidneys are rapidly excised and placed in ice-cold solution [mmol/l]: 150 K-cyclamate, 10 HEPES, 1 $CaCl_2$, 1 $MgCl_2$, pH 7.4. After decapsulation, superficial cortical slices of about 0.5 mm thickness are dissected and minced with a scalpel. Dounce homogenizer is used for tissue homogenization by three strokes with a loose-fitting pestle. The homogenate is then poured through graded sieves (250, 75 and 40 μm) to obtain a population of single cells. Light microscopy is used for identification of cells, by long microvilli distributed over the entire cell surface and can easily be distinguished from remaining erythrocytes, cell detritus and tubular fragments.

(b)   Diuretic activity in rats (Lipschitz test, *in vivo* method)

Background: This method was described by Lipschitz et al. in 1943. It is based on water and sodium excretion in test animals and compared to rats (control group) treated with a high dose of urea.

Requirements: Male Wistar rats (160–200 g), urea, sodium chloride, flame photometer, hydrochlorothiazide.

Methodology

Animals are divided into two groups and each group contains three animals. Three animals per group are placed in metabolic cages provided with a wire mesh bottom and a funnel to collect the urine. It should be equipped with stainless-steel sieves over funnel to retain feces and to allow the urine to pass. Animals are given free access to water and feed before experiment. However, food and water are withdrawn fifteen hours prior to the experiment.

Administration of drug: The test compound is administered orally at a dose of (50 mg/kg) in 5.0 ml water/kg body weight.

Induction of diuresis: 1 g/kg urea orally is given in addition to this, 5 ml of 0.9% NaCl solution per 100 g body weight are given by gavage.

Recording: Urine excretion is recorded after 5 h and after 24 h. The sodium content of the urine is determined by flame photometry.

Evaluation: Urine volume excreted per 100 g body weight is calculated for each group.

Calculation: Results are expressed as the "Lipschitz-value", i.e., the ratio T/U, in which T is the response of the test compound, and U, that of urea treatment. Calculating this index for the 24 h excretion period as well as for 5 h indicates the duration of the diuretic effect.

Note:

- Similar to urine volume, quotients can be calculated for sodium excretion.

- Indices of 1.0 and more are regarded as a positive effect. With potent diuretics, Lipschitz values of 2.0 and more can be found. Saluretic drugs, like hydrochlorothiazide, show Lipschitz values around 1.8.

(c) Saluretic activity in rats

Background: Saluretic activity is important to treat edema, ascites in congestive heart failure and hypertension. Saluretic activity refers to excretion of sodium but potassium must be sparinged.

Requirements: Albino rats (120-220 g)

Methodology: Animals are fed with standard diet and given free access to water. Food is deprived before 24 h. Test compounds are administered in a dose of 50mg/kg orally in 0.5 ml/100g body weight starch suspension. 3 animals are kept in one metabolic cage to collect urine. Animals are divided into 2 groups each containing 1 cage. Urine excretion is measured every hour. With the help of flame photometer sodium and potassium level is checked.

10.2 Uricosuric and Hypouricemic Activity

(a) Inhibition of xanthine oxidase (hypouricemic activity; *in vitro* study)

Xanthine oxidase is an iron molybdenum flavoprotein (FAD) and it contains two iron-sulfer centers.

Background: Xanthine oxidase converts hypoxanthine to xanthine and further to uric acid. This step is inhibited by allopurinol. The concentration of uric acid which gets converted from the substrate (xanthine) is determined by UV spectrometry.

Requirements: Incubator, EDTA, phosphate buffer, xanthine

Methodology:

The test compound is incubated with xanthine oxidase, EDTA and phosphate buffer solution (pH 7.8) at 37 °C. Xanthine can be determined by measuring the change in optical density in the UV range (293nm).

(b) Hypouricemic activity after allantoxanamide treatment in rats (*in vivo* study)

Background: Allantoxanamide treatment increases serum uric acid in rats. Experimental hyperuricemia can be induced by inhibition of the enzyme uricase. Uricase catalyzes uric acid to allantoin. Allantoxanamide inhibits uricase and increases endogenously synthesized uric acid. This increase is blocked by compounds like allopurinol.

Requirement: Male Sprague Dawley rats/ Wistar rats (150-220 g), allantoxanamide, allopurinol

Methodology

Eight rats are used for the each dose of test drugs and standard. Hyperuricemia is induced by allantoxanamide administration (250 mg/kg, i.p.) suspended in 5ml/kg seasame oil. The test compound is given orally in a dose of 50 mg/kg in 40 ml/kg water. Standard compound allopurinol is given in a dose of 50 mg/kg.

Urine collection: Urine is collected after drug administration of 1 to 6 h and 7 to 24 h.

Blood collection: Blood is withdrawn by retro-orbital vein puncture prior and 2, 6 and 24 h after test and standard drug administration.

Determination of uric acid: Uric acid is determined with the Uric-aquant-method in plasma and urine in mmol/l.

Evaluation: Mean values of uric acid concentrations in plasma at the different time intervals and mean values of uric acid excretion after 6 and 24 h of the test group are compared with the control group (allantoxanamide treated only) using Student's t-test.

(c) Phenolsulfonphthalein excretion in rats (*in vivo* study)

Background: Phenolsulfonphthalein (Phenol red) excretion test is used for uricosuric activity. Phenol red is mainly eliminated by active secretion in the proximal tubulus of the kidney. Uricosuric agents decrease the secretory activity of tubule cells which in turn leads to delayed excretion of phenol red.

Requirements: Male Wistar rats/ Sprague Dawley Rats (150-180 g), phenolsulfonphthalein, saline, sodium chloride, sodium carbonate, spectrophotometer.

Methodology

30 minutes before the test animals are treated with the test compound (orally) 2.5 ml/kg of a 3% aqueous solution of phenol red is administered through intravenous injection via the tail vein. Blood samples are collected after 30, 60 and 180 min via retro orbital puncture.

Sampling of blood: 0.2 ml of blood is diluted with 2 ml 0.9% NaCl-solution and centrifuged. To 1 ml of the supernatant 1 ml of 1% sodium carbonate solution and 8 ml of saline are added. Using spectrophotometer extinction values are determined at 546 nm. Extinction values are calculated for total blood.

10.3 Impaired Renal Function

(a) Chronic renal failure in the rat

Background: This animal model was described by Acott et al. in 1987. Chronic renal failure is frequent pathological condition in man having value to screen new diuretics drug.

Requirements: Sprague-Dawley rats, anesthetics (ketamine and droperidol/fentanyl)

Methodology

In rats through a 6 cm midline incision in the abdominal wall the small bowel and cecum are lifted and placed on saline-soaked gauze sponges. The exposed right kidney is dissected from the retroperitoneal area and the vascular and ureteric pedicles are ligated with silk sutures, transacted, and the kidney is removed.

Exposure of renal artery: The renal artery of the left kidney is dissected into the hilum to expose the three main segmental renal arteries. The kidney is not dissected out of the peritoneum. The anterior caudal branch of the artery is then temporarily ligated to establish the volume of renal tissue supplied.

Ligation: The area of ischemia becomes demarcated within 10-15 s. If this approximates 25% to 33% of the kidney, a permanent ligature is placed.

Closure of skin:

In the abdomen, the viscera is then carefully removed, and the peritone um and linea alba are covered with a continuous suture. The skin is co vered with clips made throughout stainless steel.

Collection of blood and urine: Serum creatinine level in blood is determined by retro-orbital puncture under anesthesia at various time intervals up to 12 months. However, creatinine, protein and specific gravity are determined in 24 h urine collection.

Evaluation

- Serum creatinine increases up to 500 μM/l after 12 months, whereas creatinine clearance decreases.
- Significantly increased urine volumes are accompanied by decreased urine specific gravity indicating a decreased concentrating ability.
- Proteinuria is significantly increased.
- Terminal uremia occurs after 14-15 months.

(b) Cisplatin induced Acute Renal Failure (ARF)

Background: Cisplatin is an anticancer agent. Cisplatin induces renal toxicity so its use is obsolete now a day. Oxidative stress, inflammation, genotoxic damage, and cell cycle arrest are responsible for its nephrotoxicity.

Requirements: Wistar rats 150-200 g or Albino mice 25-30 g, cisplatin.

Methodology:

Induction of ARF: ARF is induced by administration of cisplatin. In mice cisplatin is administered at a dose of (7 mg/kg, i.p.) and in rats (3 mg/kg, i.p.). Kidney failure starts after 2nd day and reaches a maximum after 3rd and 4th day depending on the doses.

Biochemical analysis of serum creatinine, urea, and uric acid levels are estimated using commercially available diagnostic kits. Tissue homogenates are analysed for myeloperoxidase (MPO), TNF-α, NFkB, and interleukins.

(c) Glycerol induced renal failure

Background: Glycerol causes renal failure by inducing ischemia, myoglobin-mediated nephrotoxicity, and cytokine released renal activities following rhabdomylosis.

Requirements: Wistar rats (150-180 g), 50% glycerol

Methodology

Experimental arrangement: Food and water are not given to animals 24 h before administration of glycerol, after which they are sacrificed for assessment of kidney function.

Glycerol is administered at a dose of (8 ml/kg, i.m.). Glycerol induces renal failure at this dose. The rats are dehydrated 18 h prior induction of myoglobinuric renal injury and sacrificed 48 h after injection of hypertonic glycerol without any restriction of diet or water.

Serum of rats is isolated 24 hours after glycerol administration and serum concentrations of BUN, creatinine, sodium and potassium are estimated as renal function indices. Myoglobine, gama glutamyl transferase and alkaline phosphatase levels are also measured.

References

- Rees, D. A., Alcolado, J.C. Animal models of diabetes mellitus. Diabet Med. 2004; 22 (4): 359-370.
- Sharma, R., et. al. Experimental models on diabetes: A comprehensive review. IJAPS. 2013; 4 (1) : 01-08.

- Srinivasan K, Ramarao P. Animal models in type 2 diabetes research: An overview. IJMR. 2007; 125 (3) : 451-472.

- Etuk, E. U. Animals models for studying diabetes mellitus. ABJNA. 2007; 125 (3) : 451-472.

- Vogel, G. H., 2002. Drug Discovery and evaluation: Pharmacological assays. Springer-verlag berlin Heidelberg publication. New York; pp. 209-227.

- Gupta, S. K., 2004. Drug screening methods. Jaypee brothers medical publishers LTD.New Delhi; pp. 236-246.

- Johns, C., Gavras, I. Models of experimental hypertension in mice. Hypertension. 1996; 28 (6): 1064-1069.

- Badyal, D. K., Lata, H., Dadhich, A. P. Animal Models of hypertension and effect of drugs. Indian J Pharmacol. 2003; 35 (6): 349-362.

- Goldstein, J. L., Brown, M. S. The LDL receptor locus and the genetics of familiar hypercholesterolemia. Annu. Rev. Genet.1979; 13:258-289.

- Brown, M. S., Goldstein, J. L. Familial hypercholesterolemia: Model for genetic receptor disease. Med Clin N Amer.1979; 73:163-20.

Chapter 11

Miscellaneous

11.1 Antiulcer Activity

Gastric ulcer is mainly caused by two factors, aggressive factor and defensive factor. Aggressive factors include acid, pepsin and *H.pylori*. Defensive factor include prostaglandin, bicarbonate and mucus. The principal stimuli acting on the parietal cells are:

- Gastrin
- Acetylcholine
- Histamine
- Prostaglandins

(a) Aspirin induced ulcers

Background: Aspirin is a non steroidal anti-inflammatory drug which inhibits the synthesis of inflammatory mediators like prostaglandins. Prostaglandins are defensive factors which shields the gastric mucosa by producing leukotrienes and bicarbonate ions. Aspirin produces mucosal damage by inhibiting the synthesis of prostaglandins.

Requirements: Albino rats (150-200 g), 2% gum acacia, ether and microscope.

Methodology: Animals are classified into two groups, with six animals each. The test drug (p.o with 2% gum acacia solution) is administered half an hour before aspirin administration. Aspirin is given at the dose of 200 mg/kg to induce ulcer. Rats are sacrificed after 4 hours of aspirin administration and their stomachs are dissected and opened with greater curvature for gastric lesion determination.

Ulcer index (UI): The index of ulcer is determined by the number of ulcers per animal and the severity scored by microscopic examination of the ulcers with the help of 10x lens and scoring are done as described in Table 11.1.

Table 11.1

Scoring	Condition of stomach
0	Normal stomach
0.5	Red coloration
1	Spot ulcers
1.5	Haemorrhagic streaks
2	Ulcer>3mm but<5mm
3	Ulcer>5mm

Calculation: Ulcer index: $U_I = U_N + U_S + U_P \times 10^{-1}$

Where, U_N = Average number of ulcer per animal

U_S = Average of severity score

U_P = Percentage of animals with ulcer

Percentage protection

$$\% \text{ protection} : \frac{(\text{Ulcer index}) \text{ control} - (\text{Ulcer index}) \text{ test}}{(\text{Ulcer index}) \text{ control}}$$

(b) Ethanol induced ulcers

Background: Alcohol increases the secretion of gastric juices and decreases mucosal resistance, so long term consumption of ethanol may lead to peptic ulcer. It mainly weakens mucosal resistance of gastric mucosa.

Requirements: Albino rats (150-200g), 99% alcohol, ether.

Methodology

Animals are classified into the different groups, with six animals each. Animals are given test drugs after 60 min of alcohol (1 ml/200g, orally) administration. Rats are sacrificed by using ether as anesthetic after 60 min. For the determination of ulcers a broad incision is made on the stomach of rats with greater curvature. Ulcer index may be calculated as formula discussed under aspirin induced ulcer.

(c) Pylorus ligation in rats

Background: Gastric juice gets accumulated in rats whose pylorus has been ligated and it causes gastric ulcer.

Requirements: Albino rats (150-200g), ether.

Methodology

Animals are fasted for 48 hours before surgery, but free access of water and single caged is permitted primarily to avoid the coprophagy [coprophagy refers to many kinds of feces-eating, including eating feces of other species (heterospecifics), of other individuals (allo-coprophagy), or one's own (auto-coprophagy)]. Animal is anaesthetized with ether and incision is made on abdomen inside the xiphoid process. Pylorus is lifted out and ligated, it covers the stomach and the abdominal wall is sutured.

Administration of drugs: Test compound is administered to the rats either orally or subcutaneously and placed in plastic cylinders. Animals are sacrificed after 20 h of pyloric ligation and the stomach dissected out.

Dissection: For the determination of ulcers a broad incision is made on the stomach with greater curvature.

Calculation: Ulcer index may be calculated as formula showing below.

Type 0: No visible ulceration

Type 1: superficial mucosal ulcer

Type 2: deep ulcers

Type 3: perforated ulcer

(d)   Histamine induced ulcer

Background: Histamine increases gastric acid secretion and prolonged acid secretion leads to peptic ulcer. Histamine is widely used for production of peptic ulcer and used to screen drugs for ulcer.

Requirements: Guinea pig (300-380 g)

Methodology: Animals are starved for 36 h with free access of water. Histamine is administered at a dose of (50 mg/kg, i.p). Promethazine hydrochloride is injected before and after histamine administration to prevent its toxicity. Test drug is administered half an hour before the histamine injection. Animals are sacrificed after 4 hours and their stomach is removed out and degree of ulceration is determined as discussed under pylorus ligation.

(e)   Acetic acid induced gastric ulcer

Background: Acetic acid induces ulceration by damaging the gastric mucosal barrier. This model has now emerged to screen antiulcer drugs.

Requirements: Albino rats of either sex (180-200 g)

Methodology: 0.05ml of acetic acid is injected into the sub mucosal layer of stomach and it produces ulcer.

(f) Perfused rat stomach preparation

Background: Ghosh and Schild (1958) introduced a method for continuous recording of acid secretion in rat. The acid secretion can be stimulated by histamine, acetylcholine and gastrin, which is effectively blocked by antiulcer drugs.

Requirements: Male Sprague Dawley or Wistar rats (180-200 g), 25% urethane solution, N/4000 sodium hydroxide, pentagastrin, histamine hydrochloride, Carbachol.

Methodology

Animals are starved overnight with supply of water *ad libitum*. Minimum four rats are used per dose of the test drug or the standard.

Anaesthesia: The animals are anaesthetized with 25 % urethane solution (0.6 ml/100 g, i.m).

Temperature: Body temperature is artificially stabilized by means of a heating pad using a rectal thermometer.

Cannulation: The trachea is exposed and cannulated for artificial respiration. The external jugular vein is exposed and cannulated with polythene tubes levelled at the tip.

Incision: The abdomen is then opened through a midline incision; pyloric end of the stomach is exposed and cannulated.

Insertion of tube: A flexible polythene tube is passed down the oesophagus and tied in the cervical region.

Washing: The stomach is washed out thoroughly by passing distilled water through the tube and allowing it come out of the pyloric cannula.

Perfusion: The stomach is then perfused continuously at a uniform rate (1 ml/min) with N/4000 sodium hydroxide. The concentration of sodium hydroxide may be adjusted so that the perfusate under basal conditions has a pH of 6.0 to 6.5.

Recorder: Changes in the acid secretion are recorded as changes in pH in response to secretogogues like pentagastrin, histamine and carbachol etc.

Induction: Gastric secretion is stimulated by continuous intravenous infusion of 100 µg/kg/h of pentagastrin or 3 mg/kg/h of histamine hydrochloride or 30 µg/kg/h of carbachol.

Administration of drug: The drug under investigation is injected either prior to each intravenous dose of a secretogogue or after acid secretion reaches a plateau following the intravenous infusion of a secretogogue.

Calculation: The inhibition of acid secretion is compared with the response of a standard antisecretory drug.

Determination of acidity: The gastric content volume is measured. After centrifugation free and total values are determined for acidity by titration with 0.1 N NaOH to pH 3.5 using Toepfer's reagent and to pH 8.0 using phenolphthalein as indicator, respectively.

Calculation: Ulcer index, volume of gastric contents and acidity of the gastric content of treated animals are compared with the controls. Using different doses, dose response curves are established for ulcer formation and gastric acid secretion.

11.2 Anti Inflammatory Activity

Inflammation is characterized by 4 symptoms i.e. rubor, calor, tumor and dolor. Inflammation is of 3 types acute, subacute and chronic. Inflammation has three characteristic phases: the first step is caused by an increase in vascular permeability leading to the exudation of blood fluid into the interstitial space, the second by infiltration of leukocytes from the blood into the tissues and the third by the development of granuloma. There are various models to screen anti-inflammatory drugs, and it mainly depends on type of inflammation.

(a) **Ultraviolet B erythema in guinea pigs**

Background: Erythema is the sign of inflammation and this sign is used to screen anti-inflammatory compounds.

Requirements: Guinea pig (200-300 g), Ultraviolet light (180-200 nm)

Methodology: Before exposure to ultraviolet rays, test drug is administered to the guinea pigs. Guinea pigs are exposed to ultraviolet rays (180-200 nm) and erythema is produced after 2 h of exposure of ultraviolet radiation. Vasodilator activity of inflammation can be measured by this model.

UV exposure: The guinea pigs are placed in a leather cuff with a hole of 1.5 × 2.5 cm, allowing the ultraviolet radiation to reach only this area. Following a 2 min ultraviolet exposure, the remaining half of the test compound is administered.

Scoring: The erythema is scored 2 and 4 h after exposure. The followings scores are given:

0 = no erythema,

1 = weak erythema,

2 = strong erythema,

4 = very strong erythema.

Evaluation: ED_{50} values can be calculated.

(b) Carrageenan- induced paw edema in rats

Background: Carrageenan induces edema which is also a sign of inflammation and it is used to screen anti-inflammatory drugs. Paw edema in rat is depicted in [Figure 11.1].

Requirements: Sprague-   Dawley/Wistar   rats   (150-250   g), carrageenan.

Methodology:

1% w/v carragenan suspension is administered to rats into subplantar region of hind paw [Figure 11.1] Left paw serves as drug treated group while right paw serves as control group. Test drug is administered 30 min before carragenan injection. Paw volume is measured. Edema is calculated with the formula

% reduction in edema =

$$\frac{\text{mean edema in carrageenan group} - \text{mean edema in drug treated group}}{\text{mean edema in carrageenan group}} \times 100$$

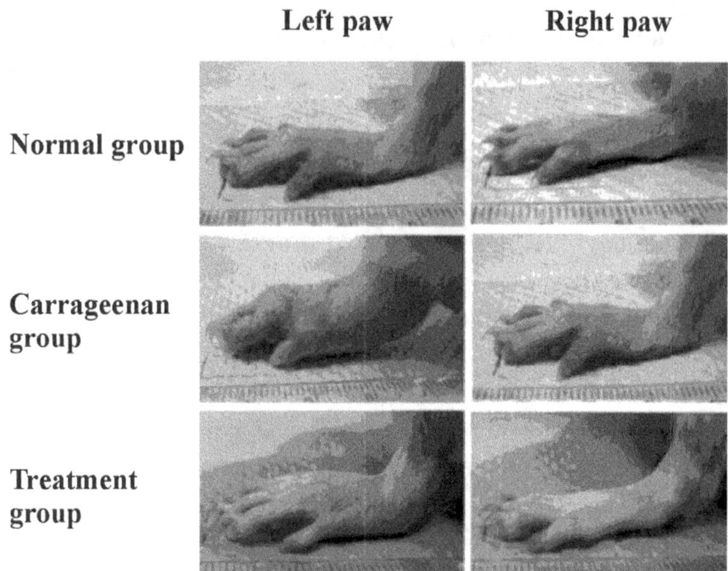

Figure 11.1 Paw edema in rat.

(c) Croton-oil ear edema in mice

Background: The source of croton oil seeds are *Croton tigilum*. It induces ear edema in mice. This model is used to detect the activity of topical anti-inflammatory drugs. Ear edema is shown in [Figure 11.2].

Requirements: Albino mice, Croton oil, Acetone, Indomethacin

Methodology: 2% of croton oil (75 µl) is administered to inner surface of left ear with 15µl of acetonic solution. Nothing is applied to the right ear. Indomethacin (100µg) is used as reference compound and control group is only applied with croton oil. Various doses of test solution may be applied to inner surface of ear [Figure 11.2]. Animals are sacrificed after 6 h and plug is removed from all the groups of animals. The difference in weight between the two plugs is measured as edema value.

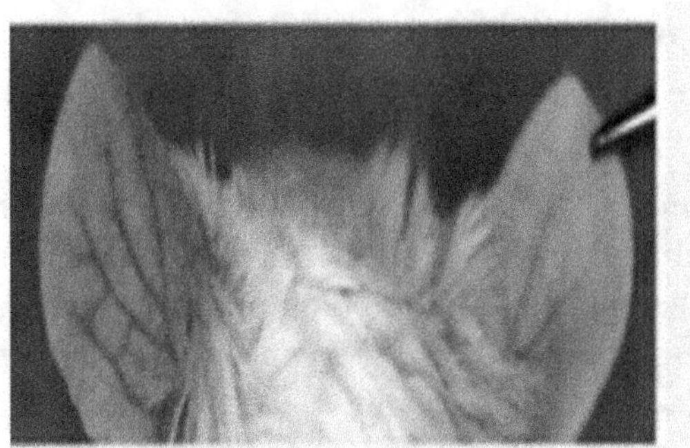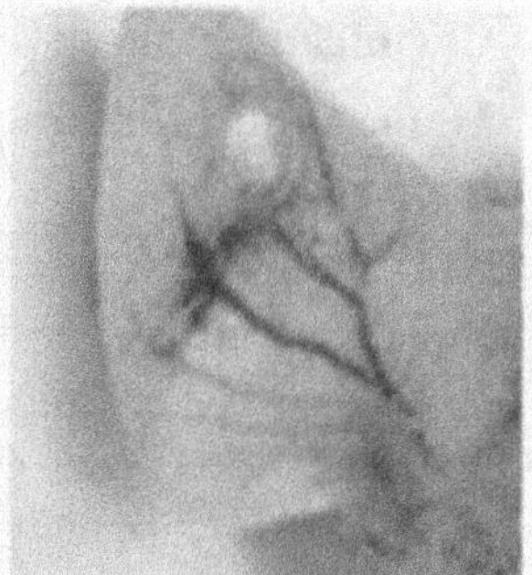

Figure 11.2 Ear edema.

11.3 Antiobesity Activity

Obesity is having too much body fat. It is multifactorial disorder and arises from the interaction between among numerous behavioral, environmental and genetic factors and associated with the dysregulation of energy homeostasis normally maintained by the hypothalamic neurotransmitter network. Signaling factors such as leptin and various neuropeptides are involved in regulating body weight. Food intake, body weight, adipose tissue cell size number, body composition, locomotor activity, plasma lipids, insulin and glucose level are studied in the animal models of obesity.

(a) Diet induced obesity

Background: The animal obesity model has been either of spontaneous or natural origin or the result of experimental manipulation of the diet.

Requirment: Albino rats (150-230 g), high fat diet.

Methodology: Adult male rats are housed individually in cages under the controlled temperature and light/dark cycle. Animals are divided in two groups. First group receives ordinary diet and other group is given in addition to chow, a high fat diet, sweetened condensed milk and number of supermarket foods like cookies, cheese, milk, chocolate pea nut butter etc. Body weight, food intake, locomotor activity, and serum insulin level are measured and compared in both the groups. After 3 months rats are sacrificed by decapitation, the number of cell sizes of adipose tissue, body composition and plasma lipids are determined and comparison is made in between the groups.

(Note: Diet may be of different varieties hyperlipidic (soyabean oil), hypercaloric (peanut, milk chocolate, and corn biscuits), cafeteria diet (biscuits, butter, cheese, and bacon), and cholesterol rich diet (cholesterol and cholic acid).

(b) Chemically induced hypothalamic obesity

Monosodium glutamate (MSG) induced hypothalamic obesity in mice and rats:

Background: Monosodium glutamate administration to newborn rats and mice causes the damage to the ventromedial hypothalamic and arcuate nuclei, leading the animals to develop obesity due to the lack of control between absorption and energy expenditure. The real mechanism by which this hypothalamic injury leads to obesity is not known.

Methodology: During neonatal age in both mice and rats monosodium glutamate is administered. In mice the dose of MSG is 2 mg/kg/body weight. MSG is administered at early stage of life for 5 consecutive days. In control group, only saline is administered. Body weight, food consumption are recorded daily. In rats dose of monosodium glutamate is 2-6mg/kg/body weight. Control group is only treated with saline. Body weight and food consumption are recorded daily.

(c) Genetic models of obesity

Monogenic models: yellow obese mouse, diabetes mouse, fat mouse, Zucker fatty rat.

Polygenic models: Japanese KK mouse, New Zealand obese (NZO) mouse.

Yellow obese mouse: In this mouse, obesity is inherited as a dominant gene. The gene is located in chromosome 2 at a linkage group 5. This mice was discovered in 1883 by Lataste and in 1905 by Cuenot.

Obese mouse: Obesity is inherited as an autososmal recessive mutation on chromosome 6. It was first discovered by Ingalls in 1950.

Diabetes mouse: Diabetes mouse was derived from mutation in C57BL/6J strain on chromosome 4. It is also an autosomal recessive mutation.

Fat mouse: Obesity is inherited an autosomal recessive mutation on chromosome 8. This mutation is known as fat mutation.

Zucker fatty rat: Zucker fatty rat is an autosomal recessive mutation. Mutation is also known as fa mutation, it was discovered by Zucker and Zucker in 1961.

Japanese KK mouse: Japanese KK mouse was discovered by Konello in Japan. Dominant gene for yellow obesity has also been transferred into the Japanese KK strain. The animals with gene for yellow obesity was referred as KK mice.

NZO mouse: NZO mouse was first described in 1953 by Bielshowsky and Bielshowsky. NZO mouse develops 50-70 g weight within 6-8 months.

11.4 Local Anesthetic Activity

Local anesthetic causes reversible loss of pain sensation. It is a reversible blocker of nerve impulses in a restricted area of the body.

(a) Conduction of anesthesia in the sciatic nerve of frog

Background: In this method head of the frogs are separated from the body and the upper part of the spinal cord is cracked down to the level of the third vertebra.

Requirements: Healthy frog, anaesthesia, 0.65% NaCl solution.

Methodology

Frog is hanged on a vertical board and viscera are removed exposing the lumbar plexus using suitable anaesthesia. White cotton balls are dipped in test preparations (0.05-1.0%) or standard and placed gently around the sciatic nerve for 1 min. Then the cotton swab is removed and the frog is placed with its extremities into a bath with 0.65% NaCl solution.

The frog is removed from the bath every three minutes and the toes of the legs or ankle joint are pinched with a small forceps three times. The reflex contraction is abolished when conduction anaesthesia is effective.

Evaluation: The time of onset and duration of anaesthesia are recorded for each concentration. The result can be presented as time response and dose response curves. For each concentration the starting time and period of anesthesia are registered. The effect can be viewed as the reaction times and dose curves.

(b) Infiltration anesthesia in guinea pigs

Background: The method of intracutaneous wheals in guinea pigs for the assessment of local anesthetic activity of novel compounds has become one of the standard procedures for the evaluation of local anesthetics.

Requirements: Guinea pigs of either sex (250-350 g), pin.

Methodology

Animal treatment: A day before experiments two areas of 4-5 cm diameter are shaved on the skin at the back of the animals.

Administration of test compound: The test and standard drugs are administered intracutaneously/through the intracutaneous route in 0.1 ml saline. This causes formation of wheal which is marked with ink.

Protocol performance: The reaction to pin prick is tested 5 min after the injection. First the normal reaction of the animal to pin prick is noted outside the wheal, later on six pricks are then applied every 5 min for 30 min inside the wheal and the number of pricks to which animal fails to react is counted.

Evaluation: The number of times the prick fails to elicit a response during the period is added up, and the cumulative number of non-responsive towards pricks give an indication of the degree of anesthesia.

Calculation: Dose response curves can be established by using a various doses.

Note: This test has been used for studying the influences of vasoconstrictors like adrenaline on the intensity and duration of action of local anesthetics.

(c) Abolition of sneezing reflex in rabbits

Background: Sneezing reflex in response to stimulation of the nasal mucosa has been used for the evaluation of local anesthetic activity.

Requirements: New Zealand albino rabbits (3-3.5 kg), cotton swab, lead pencil.

Methodology

Administration of test drug: The test solution is applied to the mucous membrane of one of the nostrils with the help of cotton swab. The standard drug solution is similarly applied to the nasal mucosa of the other nostril.

Stimulation: After 2-5 min the nasal mucous membrane is stimulated by the fine tip of a sharpened lead pencil.

Protocol Performance: Loss of sneezing reflex is considered as the sign of complete local anesthesia. The stimulation is repeated after 3, 5, 10 and 15 min and continued every 5 min until the sneezing reflex reappears.

Evaluation: The time required for the onset of action and the duration of anesthetic effects are noted using various concentrations of test compounds and the standard.

11.5 Anticancer Activity

Cancer is characterized by uncontrolled division of cells that have transformed from the normal cells to cancerous cells of the body. The cancer cells can invade the nearby cells and distant tissues via the circulation. Anticancer medicines have been produced from a variety of sources, ranging from natural products to synthetic molecules. The major side effect of anticancer drugs are bone marrow suppression, alopecia, nausea, vomiting. Therefore anticancer drugs or molecules must be identified which can be of therapeutic value in human cancers. Many chemicals are carcinogens. These chemicals are used to induce cancer in animal models. Carcinogens get metabolized and activated to induce carcinogenesis. Various screening methods are described below

(a) **DMBA-induced mouse skin papillomas (7, 12-Dimethylbenz [a] anthracene)**

Background: This is a classical two stage experimental carcinogenesis model. Mouse skin is generally most sensitive to epidemic carcinogenesis.

Requirements: Swiss albino mice of either sex, DMBA.

Methodology: DMBA acts as an initiator and 12-O-tetradecanpoyl-phorbol-13-acetate (TPA) are used as a promoter to induce skin papillomas and squamous cell carcinomas. Mice are topically applied with a single dose of 2.5 µg DMBA in acetone on the shaved back, followed by 5-10 µg of TPA in 0.2 ml acetone twice daily on the same site starting one week after DMBA application. Papillomas begin to appear after 6-7 weeks of application of TPA. Tumor development is weekly monitored till the experiments terminate after 18 weeks. Percent tumor incidence and multiplicity of treatment group is compared with DMBA control group.

(b) N-methyl, N- nitrosourea (MNU) - induced rat mammary gland carcinogenesis

Background: N-Methyl-N-nitrosourea (MNU) is a direct-acting alkylating agent that interacts with DNA. Accumulation of mutations can increase the risk of cancer in the target organs or cause cell death in susceptible tissues or cells if excessive damage to DNA is not repaired.

Reqirments: Wistar albino rats (250-350 g), MNU

Methodology: Single intravenous administration of 50 mg/kg body weight of MNU (pH 5.0) is administered in rats. The tumors produced in this model are 75-95% within 180 days. MNU-induced tumors are invasive and predominantly adenocarcinomas. This model is the better model for human breast cancer.

(c) Azoxymethane (AOM)-induced aberrant crypt foci in rat

Background: Aberrant crypt foci are single and multiple colonic crypts containing cells exhibiting dysplasia. These are potential precancerous lesions and are being evaluated as intermediate biomarkers for colon cancer in rodents.

Requirement: Albino rats (150-250 g), AOM

Methodology: Aberrant crypt foci can be produced by a single injection of 30 mg AOM /kg body weight in rats. Drug treatment schedule can vary depending on the selection. At the end of the treatment, animals are sacrificed, and frequencies of aberrant crypt foci are determined by histopathologic examination.

(d) N-Butyl-N (4-hydroxybutyl)-nitrosamine (OH-BBN)-induced bladder carcinoma in mouse

Background: OH-BBN induces urinary bladder invasive transitional cell carcinomas that are morphologically similar to that of the human variant of advanced urinary bladder transitional cell carcinomas.

Requirement: Male BDF mice of fifty days old, OH-BBN.

Methodology: 7.5 mg of OH-BBN is intra-gastrically instilled till 8 weeks from beginning at fifty days of age. Drug effectiveness is measured as percent reduction in the incidence of transitional cell carcinoma compared with carcinogen control group. This model induces about 40% tumor incidence during 180 days of experimental period in control animals.

References

- Rees, D. A., Alcolado, J.C. Animal models of diabetes mellitus. Diabet Med. 2004 ; 22 (4): 359-370.

- Sharma, R., et. al. Experimental models on diabetes: A comprehensive review. IJAPS. 2013; 4 (1): 01-08.

- Srinivasan K, Ramarao P. Animal models in type 2 diabetes research: An overview. IJMR. 2007; 125 (3): 451-472.

- Etuk, E. U. Animals models for studying diabetes mellitus.ABJNA. 2007; 125 (3): 451-472.

- Vogel, G. H., 2002. Drug Discovery and evaluation: Pharmacological assays. Springer-Verlag berlin Heidelberg publication. New York; pp. 209-227.

- Gupta, S. K., 2004. Drug screening methods. Jaypee brothers medical publishers LTD. New Delhi; pp. 236-246.

- Johns, C., Gavras, I. Models of experimental hypertension in mice. Hypertension. 1996; 28 (6): 1064-1069.

- Badyal, D. K., Lata, H., Dadhich, A. P. Animal Models of hypertension and the effect of drugs. Indian J Pharmacol. 2003; 35 (6): 349-362.

- Goldstein, J. L., Brown, M. S. The LDL receptor locus and the genetics of familiar hypercholesterolemia. Annu. Rev. Genet.1979; 13:258-289.

- Brown, M. S., Goldstein, J. L. Familial hypercholesterolemia: Model for genetic receptor disease. Med Clin N Amer.1979; 73:163-20.

- Choudhary, M..K., Bodakhe, S.H, Gupta, S .K. Assessment of antiulcer potential of Moringa Oliefera root bark extract in rats. J Acupunct Meridian Stud. 2013; 6 (4): 214-220.

Chapter 12

Transgenic Animals and other Genetically Modified Animal Models

12.1 Introduction

Recombinant DNA development is the mechanism used to demonstrate foreign DNA inside the animal's body and the germ line should be transferred a short time later so that each cell, even animal germ cells, contain the same modified genetic material. An animal whose genetic structure has been deliberately altered by the development of foreign DNA is said to be transgenic, the DNA that is introduced is known as a transgene, and the general system is called transgenesis.

12.1.1 Method of Creation of Transgenic Animals

Theoretically, the procedure to accomplish this goal is clear and can be gotten by infusing the cloned gene into the nucleus of a fertilized egg, implanting the inoculated fertilized egg into a receptive female in light of the fact that successful completion of mammalian embryonic development is not possible outside of a female. The animals which indicate cloned gene incorporated into their germ line cells are then bred to set up new genetic lines. The three critical strategies utilized for the making of transgenic animals are:

(a) DNA microinjection

This method involves the direct microinjection of a chosen gene construct into the pronucleus of a fertilized ovum from another member of the same species or from another species. It is one of the first methods in mammals which have proved effective. The introduced DNA may lead to the over expression or under expression of specific genes or to the expression of completely new genes for the animal species. The manipulated fertilized ovum is transferred into the oviduct of a recipient female or fosters mother that has been induced to act as a recipient by mating with a vasectomized male (Figure 12.1).

Advantage:

- The significant advantage of this method is its applicability to a wide variety.

- DNA (genes) delivered by this technique is not constant and can be optimized.

- The delivery is precise and used for the choice of integrative transformation.

- DNA microinjection producing transgenic mice is a powerful tool for studying the molecular regulation of gene expression.

Limitation:

- The injection can cause damage that affects embryonic development and high mortalities.

- Only one cell is injected per injection.

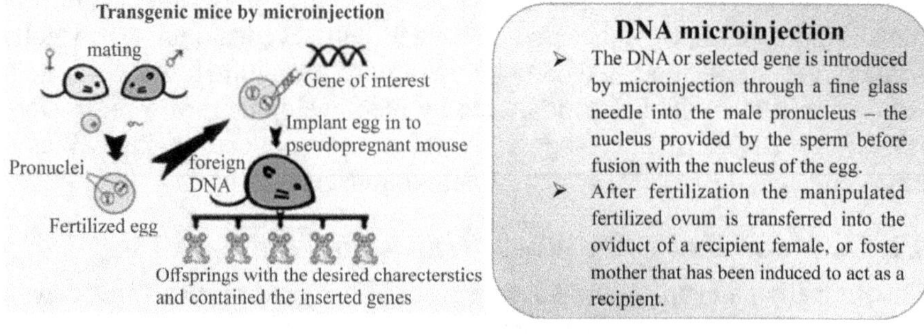

Figure 12.1 DNA microinjection.

(b) Embryonic stem cell-mediated gene transfer

This method involves prior insertion of the desired DNA sequence into an *in vitro* culture of embryonic stem cells (ES) through homologous recombination. Stem cells are undifferentiated cells that have the ability to divide into any cell type and thus give rise to an entire organism (Figure 12.2).

At the developmental stage of the blastocyst these cells are then integr ated into an embryo, results in a chimeric animal. ES cell-mediated gene transfer is the method of choice for gene inactivation, the so-called knock-out method.

Note: This approach is of particular importance for studying the genetic regulation of processes of development.

Advantage: It has the advantage of allowing precise targeting by homologous recombination of identified mutations within the gene. For mice, the technique works well.

Disadvantage: Transgenic animals sometimes may induce mutagenesis. The low survival rate of transgenic animals.

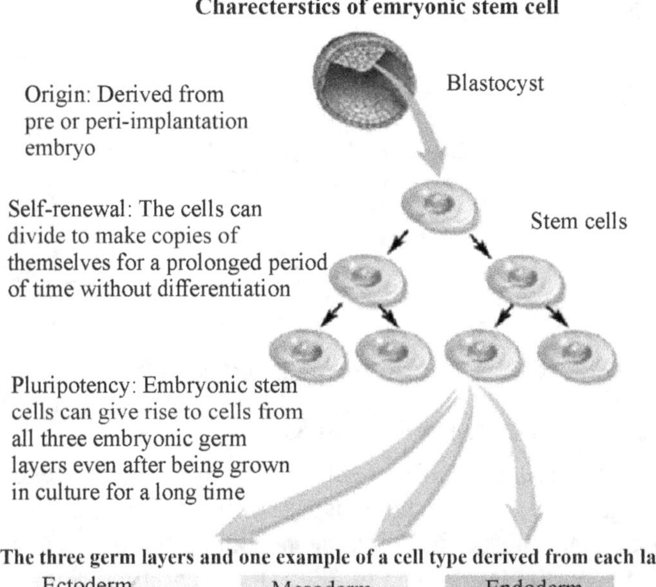

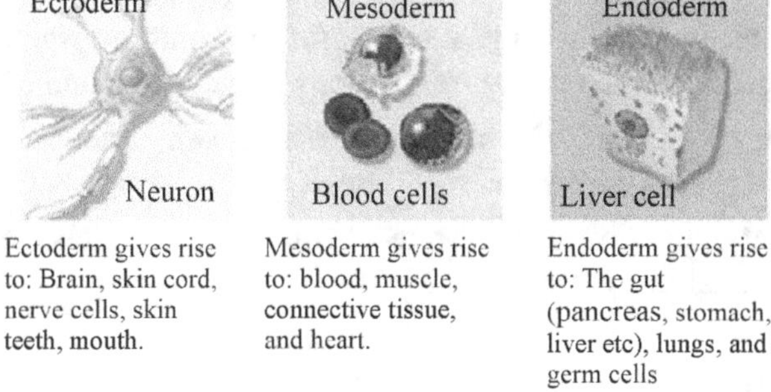

The three germ layers and one example of a cell type derived from each layer:

Ectoderm	Mesoderm	Endoderm
Ectoderm gives rise to: Brain, skin cord, nerve cells, skin teeth, mouth.	Mesoderm gives rise to: blood, muscle, connective tissue, and heart.	Endoderm gives rise to: The gut (pancreas, stomach, liver etc), lungs, and germ cells

Figure 12.2 DNA microinjection.

(c) Retrovirus-mediated gene transfer

The probability of expression increases when gene transmission is mediated through a carrier or vector. Retroviruses are widely used as vectors for the passage of genetic material into the cell, thereby benefiting from their ability to infect host cells. The offspring produced from this process is chimeric, i.e. the retrovirus is not borne by all cells. Transmission of the transgene is possible only if the retrovirus integrates into some of the germ cells (Figure 12.3).

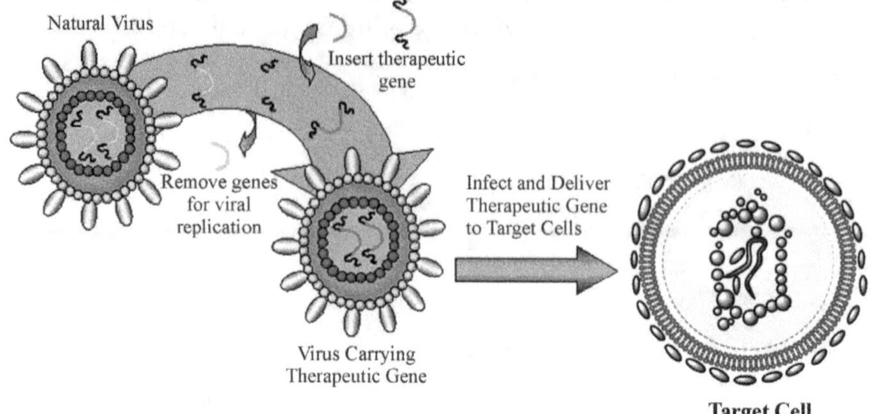

Figure 12.3 Retrovirus-mediated gene transfer.

(d) Transposon-mediated gene transfer

Transposons are DNA fragments that join with the genomes. The desired gene can replace the transposase gene of the transposons. This signifies that transposase or a gene coding for this enzyme is co-injected with the transposon to allow its integration. Transposon P is used to generate transgenic *Drosophila*. Various transgenic animals are produced with the use of transposons like chicken and Medaka etc.

Advantage: Transposons make up a significant fraction of genome and play an essential part in evolution.

Disadvantage: Low survival rate of transgenic animals, mutagenesis and functional disorder.

References

*   Houdebine, L. M. Transgenic animal models in biomedical research. Methods Mol Biol. 2007; 360:163-202.

*   Tsika, R. W. Transgenic animal models. Exerc Sport Sci Rev. 1994; 22: 361-388.

Chapter 13

Drug Toxicity and Safety Evaluation

13.1 Introduction

No drug is entirely safe; it is the dose, which differentiates between the drug and the poison. All the drugs have some intended effects and some unintended (side effect and toxic effect) effects. It is very crucial to interpret whether this benefit outweighs the risk or risk outweighs the benefit. Side effects are unavoidable and undesirable, but sometimes it may be beneficial. Adverse effects are a pharmacological extension of the drug due to overdosing or prolonged use, genetic predisposition, inappropriate use, and sometimes-non selective actions. For example coma by barbiturate, bleeding due to heparin. Adverse effects may become life-threatening.

Toxicology is mainly focused on the ill effects of drugs in the animal and human body. Safety testing and toxicity testing is essential for drug development, and this testing is done at both preclinical and clinical levels.

13.1.1 Factors Affecting Drug Toxicity

Various factors affect drug toxicity like patient age, genetic factors, pathological condition, dose, drug-drug interaction. Various types of toxicities are listed below:

(a) **Depending on the site of action**

- **On target toxicity:** It is caused by the drug, which binds to its intended receptor but at an inappropriate concentration with suboptimal concentration.

- **Off-target toxicity:** It is caused by the drug, which binds with a receptor that is not intended for it and shows a toxic reaction.

(b) **Depending on the action**

- **Cytotoxicity:** It refers to damage to the cells or specific organ by a drug or its active metabolite. For example, damage to the eyes or ears, potentially fatal loss of function of the liver.

- **Teratogenicity:** It refers to damage of embryo by teratogens. Teratogens can cross the placental barrier and affect the fetus during pregnancy at different trimester. For example, tetracycline, doxycycline, ACE inhibitors captopril, benazepril.

- **Mutagenicity:** It refers to mutation of the gene caused by some physical or chemical drugs. It affects the DNA of an organism hence the recurrence of mutation is increased for example, ionization radiation, ultraviolet radiation, alkylating drugs, transposon

- **Carcinogenicity:** It refers to certain substances, which produces cancer. Carcinogens can induce tumors (benign or malignant).

13.2 Safety Evaluation

Safety evaluation is necessary for drug development in various branches such as pharmacological parameters, toxicological parameters and it may be associated with the chemistry of the compound. Safety parameters need to be evaluated because of the presence of multiple contaminants and impurities because of growing adulteration. Before preclinical testing, the compound should be free from any kind of pollutants or impurities.

Drug safety evaluation based on this encyclopedic approach include the consideration of the following key factors :

- **Pharmacology:** Toxicity of any drug may be the result of drug-receptor interaction, interaction with the different receptor of the drug.

- **Chemistry:** Chemical structure may be responsible for drug toxicity.

- **Toxicology:** Toxicity may be because of various parameters in intact animals and in human cells culture.

- **Drug metabolism and pharmacokinetics:** Pharmacokinetic parameters such as absorption, distribution, metabolism and excretion, drug-drug interaction, these parameters are mainly responsible for drug toxicity.

- **Risk factors:** various risk factors are involved such as physiological, genetic and environmental factors. It is recommended that the drug safety and the efficiency of drug development may be increased due to this unified and interdisciplinary approach.

13.2.1 General Preclinical Safety Testing

(a) Preclinical safety testing is performed before clinical trials

It is carried out in small animals. A key component of investigational new drug (IND) application in preclinical drug development is the safety study, which gathers preliminary efficacy, toxicity, and pharmaco-kinetic data and establishes the initial dose range for the human in Phase 1 clinical trial. The objective of the preclinical safety study is to check the therapeutic and toxicity parameters before clinical trial and all over the drug development during clinical trials. Both *in vitro* and *in vivo* studies can be used for the characterization. Following factors should be considered for the preclinical safety testing.

- Selection of the proper animal species
- Age
- Physiological state
- The way of delivery, including dose, route of administration, and treatment regimen
- Test materials stability under the using conditions.

(b) Preclinical toxicity studies

Toxicity studies should be conducted in compliance with Good Laboratory Practice (GLP). In some cases, due to the lack of facility and time, full GLP compliance can not be achieved but that does not necessarily mean that we can not use the data from these studies to support clinical trials and marketing authorizations. The conventional approaches of toxicity testing of pharmaceuticals and biopharmaceuticals are not same due to the unique and diverse structural and biological properties of the later that may include specificity of the species, unpredicted pleiotropic activities, immunogenicity.

(c) Pharmacodynamics/ Biological Activity

In vitro assays can be used to evaluate the biological activity and to determine the key effects of the product which may be responsible for the clinical activity. The direct effect of the product on cellular phenotypes and proliferation can be evaluated by using cell line or by primary cell cultures. As some biopharmaceuticals have species specific action, so it is vital to select the proper animal species for the toxicity testing .

In vitro cell line culture of mammalian cells can be used to anticipate specific aspects of *in vivo* activity and to assess the relative sensitivity of various species (including human) to the biopharmaceutical quantitatively. Receptor affinity, receptor occupancy and pharmacological activity may be evaluated by such studies. Such study can also help to select proper animal species for the further *in vivo* pharmacology and toxicology study. The combined results from *in vivo* and *in vitro* studies help to extrapolate the findings to humans. The proposed use of the product in clinical studies is justified by pharmacological activity including defining mechanism of action obtained from *in vivo* study.

For monoclonal antibodies, the immunological properties of the antibody should be described in detail, including its specificity to antigen, complement binding, and any unexpected reactivity and/or cytotoxicity towards human tissues distinct from the actual target. By using a range of human tissues such cross-reactivity studies should be performed by appropriate immune histochemical procedures.

Selection of model/ animal species

Standard toxicity testing designs on commonly used species often cease due to the species specific and tissue specific biological activity.Only relevant species should be used in safety evaluation programs. In the relevant species the test material is pharmacologically active due to the expression of the receptor or an epitope (in the case of monoclonal antibodies). A relevant species can be identified by a number of techniques (e.g., functional and immunochemical tests).

One should have knowledge about receptor/epitope distribution to understand potential *in vivo* toxicity.

One animal species can be considered as relevant animal species for testing of monoclonal antibodies which express the desired epitope and shows a cross-reactivity profile similar to human tissues. Thus expression of the desired epitope will increase the ability to evaluate the toxicity arising from the binding and any unintentional cross reactivity. The animal species which does not have the expression of the particular epitope may be relevant for assessing toxicity if comparable unintentional tissue cross reactivity to humans is demonstrated.

13.3 Clinical Safety Testing

An investigational new drug (IND) application must be submitted to FDA by the drug developing company before beginning of the clinical research. In India its Central Drugs Standard Control Organization (CDSCO), the drug controller general of India (DCGA) gives approval of new drugs and clinical trails. There are 4 phases in a clinical trial.

Phase 1: The effect of the drug using different dosage form is established by using a small number of (20-50) healthy volunteers or people to avoid serious toxicity. But if it is predicted that the drug have remarkable toxicity, as in case of AIDS and cancer therapy, volunteer patients suffering from the disease are used instead of normal volunteers. Although the main aim of this study is to calculate the maximum tolerated dose and to establish the safety window in humans. Phase 1 trials are the open or non-blind type, in which both the investigators and volunteer knew what treatment is being given. Pharmacokinetic studies like absorption, metabolism, and half-life are evaluated in this phase. These studies are generally executed in the authorized research centers and hospitals by specially trained clinical pharmacologist.

Phase 2: In this clinical trial the drug is investigated in the volunteer patients having a particular disease to evaluate its therapeutic efficacy and side effects by using a modest number of (100-200) volunteer. Phase 2 of the clinical trial is a single-blind study, in which only the investigators know which treatment/placebo (or other intervention) the participants are receiving. Toxicities of the product is also evaluated in a extended range in this phase.

Phase 3: This phase is conducted on a large number of (300-3000) volunteer patients with having the particular disease to determine its efficacy and safety. Phase 3 studies are designed to minimize the errors like the variable course of the disease etc. caused by the placebo treatment, using information collected in phase 1 and phase 2 clinical trials. Therefore double blind techniques are frequently used, in which neither the participants nor the experimenters know who is receiving a particular treatment/placebo. This clinical trial can be challenging to design, execute and expensive because a large number of volunteer participation and a huge number of data is generated which must be compiled and interpreted. Some toxic effects like immunological deposition may first become apparent in this clinical trial. Specialist investigator for the particular disease should be employed.

If the company get the expected result in phase 3, they can apply for ther permission for the marketing of the new drug. To get the marketing permission, the company have to submit a New Drug Application (NDA) to the FDA. Full reports of all preclinical and clinical trials are provided in the application form. FDA may take from a month to a year to review the NDA which may lead to the approval (or denial). Preference approval is given to the drugs that represent the significant improvement as compared to the marketed drugs. FDA takes expert committees advice on drug safety, effectiveness, and labeling. Standard approval which takes longer time and designated for products judged similar to products present in the market. The whole course of preclinical, clinical and NDA review by FDA can be speeded up in case of any urgency (e.g., cancer chemotherapy, AIDS). FDA may allow controlled marketing of the new drug for serious diseases prior to the completion of phase 3 clinical studies like development of COVID 19 vaccine. Approval from the FDA is one of the critical factors in the time the drug takes to be marketed and to reach to the patients.

Phase 4: Phase 4 clinical trial starts after a drug get approval for the marketing by FDA, it is also called the post-marketing surveillance. In this phase safety of the new drug under the substantial situations are used in a large number of recipients. It evaluates the drug taken by patients under a wide range of circumstances over an extended period of time. Several thousand diseased volunteers are involved in this phase. Safety, efficacy and any other benefits have been evaluated which is the main aim of this study. The main aim of this Phase 4 is to evaluate any positive and negative effect of the drug which is undetectable previously. Post-marketing surveillance mainly deals with the detection and monitoring of adverse drug reactions (ADRs). Phase 4 clinical trial has no fixed duration.

Reference

- Riley, A. L., Kohut, S. Drug Toxicity. In: Stolerman I.P. (Eds). Encyclopedia of Psychopharmacology. Springer, Berlin, Heidelberg. 2010, pp. 29-39.

- Keysser, C. H. Preclinical safety testing of new drugs. Ann Clin Lab Sci. 1976; 6 (2): 197-205.

- Katzung, B. G. Basic and Clinical Pharmacology. McGraw-Hill Education. 2017, ISBN-13: 978-1259641152.

Chapter 14

Alternatives to Animal Screening Procedures

14.1 Introduction

Alternatives to animal screening procedures are to develop such methods which avoid live animal use. Russell and Burch in their publication, 'The Principles of Humane Animal Experimental Techniques' have developed various options for animal. They developed three 'Rs' principle as 'Reduction, Refinement and Replacement 'as substitution. Now a days it is very much popular in biomedical research.

14.1.1 Replacement

Animals can be replaced by two methods, one of which is the use of cells or tissues of animals (relative replacement) and another is the substitution method with another method, which is devoid of the using of animal(complete replacement). *In vitro* studies may be better alternative, where tissues in culture and cells are used instead of animal.

Advantage: Numbers of agent's toxicity or mutagen study can be conducted by using less expensive model.

Disadvantage: It is difficult to determine all the physiological and pathological variables in a system, compared to live animal.

Now a days forth "R" has been added, which is "Reuse". wherever possible 'reuse' of animal may be considered after approval from ethical committee.

14.1.2 Reduction

It means decreasing the animals number required to execute any experiment or to educate about any concept. Experimental design must be prepared with due care, and sophisticated statistical techniques must be used so that a lesser number of animals are used.

14.1.3 Refinement

Refinement means to make some small changes in the experimental designs to reduce pain every time whenever it is possible by the researchers. Following measures should be adopted to refine the protocol or experiment:

- Proper training must be obtained before any experimental procedure.
- Handling techniques for animals must be adequate.
- The dose of the drug should be correct, and it must not have crossed the expiry date.
- To make sure that the performed procedures on the animal are rational for the used species.
- Use of proper analgesics and antipyretics for a severe surgical procedure every time.
- The aseptic environment must be maintained to prevent any unwanted reaction during surgery.
- The post-surgical concern should be there such as to maintain the body temperature and fluid balance.

If any other test has been confirmed, then it is entirely up to the governing body to take a decision whether they are going to accept the alternative or not. There are two alternatives to substitute *in vivo* animal models, one of which is *in silico* computer simulation technique and other is *in vitro* cell culture method. Skin irritation test in human and human blood can be used for pyrogen test. Sometimes microdosing can also be useful. Now a days fourth "R" has been added, which is "Reuse". Wherever possible "reuse" of animals may be considered after approval from ethical committee.

14.2 *In Vitro* Methods

Tissue culture and cells should be used instead of animals for the screening of anti-AIDS, anti-cancer, and any other drugs. These methods are also used to study therapeutic proteins, antibiotics and vaccines.

Advantages

- Number of tests on an animal can be reduced by using tissue culture or cells.
- Serum of the animal is required be used to maintain the cells in the culture.
- Now a days, mutagenic properties of the test substances are regularly evaluated by using cell cultures.

Disadvantages

- Very much tough to get exact results.
- It is reported that over one million fetal cows are killed every year to get bovine serum which is a key component of culture medium.

14.2.1 Other Methods to Reduce Animal Involvement

- Animal-based irritative and corrosive tests can be substituted by equivalent human skin tests.

- An *in vitro* test, "Corrositex" which evaluate chemical corrosivity. That is used for rabbit's dermal corrosivity test can be replaced by this 'Corrositex' test.

14.3 *In Silico* Methods

In *in silico* method, drug testing is carried out in specific computer programs. Compounds having resembling structure shows analogous properties, so computer programs are developed in such a way, so that related structural compounds are screened simultaneously.

14.3.1 Skin Irritation and Skin Corrosion

Skin irritation and corrosion is the local toxic effects due to the local exposure of the skin to a substance. Animal-based irritative and corrosive tests can be substituted by equivalent human skin tests. Organization for Economic Co-operation and Development (OECD) introduced the new 439 test guidelines in August 2010 which consists of the detailed *in vitro* test needed to determine the hazardous nature of irritant chemicals. Test Guideline 439 consists of the detailed description of the *in vitro* tests to identify hazardous nature of irritant chemicals mixtures and substances according to the classification and labelling of Category 2 of the Globally Harmonized System of UN. This guideline instructed to use reconstructed human epidermis (RhE), which closely resembles to human epidermis physiologically and biochemically. The growth pattern of the cell is evaluated by a test, in which MTT dye enzymatically converted into formazan (blue salt) which is measured quantitatively after extraction from tissues. Test substances irritative nature are determined by considering its ability of decreasing cell growth below-specific threshold levels (below or equal to 50% for UN GHS Category 2. Colored chemicals can be evaluated by HPLC technique.

14.3.2 Phototoxicity

Phototoxicity is mainly characterized by inflammation, swelling and rash, due to the exposure to light (sun burn) following to a chemical exposure. OECD approved Neutral Red Uptake (NRU) Phototoxicity Test is used to determine the viability of 3T3 cells in the absence or presence of light after exposure to a chemical.

14.3.3 High Throughput Screening (HTS)

This is a fastest drug-discovery process which is a combination of biology, engineering, informatics and chemistry. 50000 to 100000 compounds can be screened in one week because of high throughput screening [Figure 14.3].

(a) Assay technology in HTS
- Cell growth tests (cell-based assays or phenotypic assays)
- Tissue response - targeted functional cell-based assay
- Enzyme test – biochemical

(b) Advantages of HTS
- High sensitivity (ability to detect single molecule)
- High speed (automatic system)
- Minimization of assay (micro titer plate assay)
- Low background signal
- Low complexity of assay (specific interaction)
- Reproducibility
- Economical cost

14.3.4 The Detection Method in HTS
- Mass Spectrometry
- Chromatography
- Colorimetry
- X-ray diffraction
- Microscopy
- Radioactive methods

14.3.5 Spectroscopy in HTS
- Fluorescence Spectroscopy
- Total internal reflection fluorescence (TIRF)
- Nuclear magnetic resonance (NMR)
- Absorption and luminescence spectroscopy.
- Fourier transform infrared spectroscopy (FTIR)
- Light scattering spectroscopy (LSS)

14.3.6 Chromatography in HTS
- Gas chromatography (GC)
- Thin layer chromatography
- High Performance Liquid chromatography (HPLC)
- Ion Pair Chromatography
- Reverse phase chromatography
- Hydrophobic interaction chromatography
- Affinity chromatography

14.3.7 Colorimetry in HTS

- Isothermal Titration Calorimetry (ITC)
- Differential Scanning Calorimetry (DSC)

14.3.8 Microscopy in HTS

- Scanning Tunneling Microscopy
- Atomic Force Microscopy
- Confocal Microscopy

14.3.9 Uses of HTS

(a) To screen all kind of novel biologically active compounds (libraries):

- Natural products
- Combinatorial Libraries (peptides, chemicals,etc.)
- Biological libraries

(b) To screen Microarrays such as:

- DNA chips
- RNA chips
- Protein chips

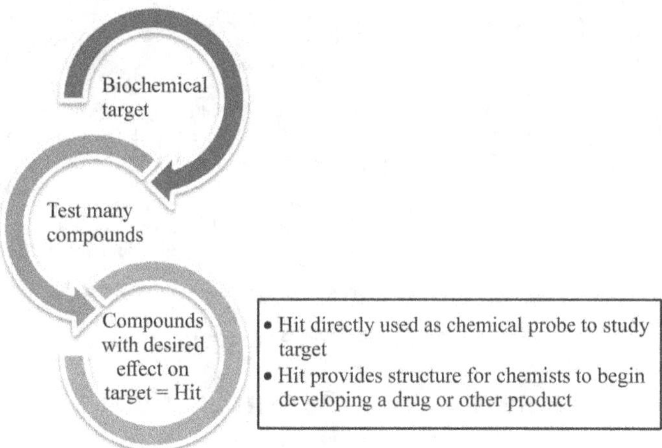

Figure 14.1 High throughput screening.

14.4 Patch Clamp Technique

Neher and Sakmann introduced this technique in 1976, and they were collectively awarded Nobel Prize for this in the year 1991. Patch clamp technique investigates about single or multiple ion channels. This technique is mainly concerned about excitable cells like neurons, cardiomyocyte and muscle fibers. It is also helpful for the study of bacterial ion channels.

14.4.1 Principle of Patch Clamp Technique

A membrane patch is removed from the cell without breaking the gigaseal. Then ion moving through the channel or ion channel opening is measured. It also monitors the current that circulates across the membrane Figure 14.2.

14.4.2 Importance of Patch Clamp Technique

- It is improvement of voltage clamp technique.
- This technique can be employed for even a single ion flowing across the membrane.
- It give access to the interior of the cell either by changing the intracellular fluid or by introducing an electrode into the cell.
- It makes an envelope impermeable to ion flow.
- It estimates current across ion channels vs voltage, time and temperature.

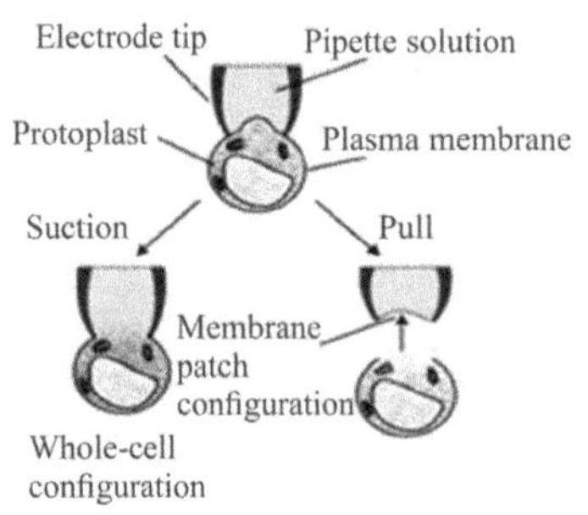

APPLICATIONS

- For the evaluation of antiarrhythmics agents.
- In kidney cells.
- Used for isolated ventricular myocytes from guinea pigs to study a cardio selective inhibition of the ATP sensitive potassium channel.
- To identify multiple types of calcium channel.
- To measure the effect of potassium channel openers.
- Used in the molecular biology.
- Voltage clamp studies on sodium channels.
- Used to investigate a wide range of electrophysiological cell properties.
- Measurement of cell membrane conductance.

Figure 14.2 Patch clamp technique.

14.5 Spectrophotometric Determination of Protein Concentration

Spectrophotometric methods are employed to evaluate the protein concentration of a sample (solution). The fluorescence technique is employed to determine the exact amount of the protein. This conventional method is used to estimate dilute protein samples. Lowry test, Bradford test, and Biuret test are used to measure the protein concentration. The process A280 is the most frequently employed method.

14.5.1 Absorbance at 280nm for Protein Estimation

Background: The principle of protein estimation at 280 nm (A280) is based on the absorption of UV light by the aromatic amino compounds in solution. The concentration of unknown protein sample is calculated by measuring the absorbance of the unknown solution at 280 nm. Then the absorbance of the unknown solution is either compared to the standard protein curve or matched with the published standard data to calculate the unknown concentration. This method can be used to quantify any solution, having the concentration ranging from 20 to 3000 µg/ml.

Requirements: Standard protein solution (3 mg/ml), unknown protein solution, UV spectrophotometer.

Methodology

- At first 3 mg/ml standard protein solution have to be prepared as stock solution from which a series of dilutions of 20, 50, 100, 250, 500, 1000, 2000, and 3000 µg/ml have to be prepared by using the same solvent which is used to prepare the sample protein solution. A blank solution also have to be prepared, consisting of only solvent.

Note: Ideally, in case of purified or partially purified protein, the standard protein should contain aromatic amino acid group same as the sample protein. Bovine serum albumin (BSA) is frequently used as standard for the spectrophotometric quantification of protein in solution. The absorbance of a 3 mg/ml BSA solution at 280 nm should be 1.98, based on an A280 of 6.61 for a 1% (w/v) solution.

- Turn on spectrophotometer's UV lamp and set the wavelength to 280 nm. Then leave, the instrument to warm up for 30 min.

- Fill the cuvette with only solvent and measure its absorbance as blank to nullify the fluctuation in the test or standard due to the absorbance of solvent.

- Take the absorbance of the standard and test protein solutions.

- Calculate the concentration of the test by using its absorbance from the given formula:

$$\text{Concentration (mg/ml)} = \frac{A280}{a280 \times b}$$

In the given formula 'a' is the absorbance of 1 mg/ml solution at 280 nm and 1 cm pathlenth and 'b' is the path length in cm.

- Prepare a calibration curve by plotting concentration at 'X' axis and A280 at 'Y' axis of the standard. Put the absorbance of the test solution of protein to find out the concentration from the calibration curve. A list of an alternative methods to animal models alongwith their advantages is given in table 14.1.

Table14.1 A List of an alternative to animal models used in biomedical research and their advantages

S. No.	Alternative models	Advantages
1.	*In vitro* studies on cell lines	1. Preparations are highly sensitive to drugs and chemicals 2. Easy to handle
2.	E-alternatives such as computer simulations, virtual laboratory environments, computer program, and virtual reality systems	1. Dissection, vivisection and technical skills can be performed over computer software without the use of animals. 2. It gives precise results without environmental and geographical hindrance. 3. The same experiment can be repeated for unlimited times. 4. It can be performed without trained demonstrator or tutor. 5. Possibility to change the drug doses and combination of drugs. 6. The demonstration can be made effective with the use of video-projector presentations, virtual conferences, and broadcasting.
3.	Models, Mannequins and Mechanical simulators	1. Useful to illustrate the topography of organs and anatomy 2. Handling of animals without animals stress and student anxiety. 3. Teaching skills like catheterization, routes of dosing and critical care in resuscitation.
4.	Film and interactive videos	1. Make learning, teaching and presentation very useful related to dissections and experiments. 2. Low cost and an unlimited number of repetitions
5.	Plant experiments such as isolation of mitochondria from plant tissue rather than obtained from a liver of a freshly killed animal	1. High sensitivity to toxic chemicals 2. Useful for studying cell respiration or electron transport from biochemistry. 3. Easy to maintain and monitor the effects.

Table 14.1 *Contd...*

S. No.	Alternative models	Advantages
6.	Waste material from slaughterhouses such as cock ileum for bioassay of drugs, eyes of goat for studying drug's effect, etc.	1. Non-invasive hands-on experience of animals and animal tissue 2. Avoid the breeding and killing of animals for tissue or organs 3. A wide range of available bodies, organs, and tissues. 4. Very cost effective as most of the tissues /organs used are picked from slaughterhouse waste.

References

- Ranganatha,N., Kuppast, J. I. A review of alternatives to animal testing methods in drug development.IJPPR. 2012; 4: 28-32.
- Bodakhe, S. H., Dangi, J. S., Ram, A., Namdeo, K. P. & Bodakhe, K. S. Isolated Cock Ileum: A Tool For Pharmacology Experiments. IJPER. 2009; 43(2), 199-202.

Chapter 15

New Approaches in Drug Discovery

15.1 Introduction

Any methodology directed towards the process of unearthing any drug and its subsequent development by the combined studies of the medical community and the pharmaceutical industry serves the goal of providing enhanced, novel and curative therapies for specific diseases. By definition, drug discovery is a complex learning process in which research efforts are directed towards the development and assimilation of new knowledge to create and develop a drug to provide benefits to a defined patient population. As a result, a highly alluring technology or strategy to drug discovery should facilitate both practical learning and the utilization of newly discovered observations that can be exploited for therapeutic benefit. However, some believe that the design of drugs is widely achieved by serendipity and, therefore, is adequately addressed by the selection of a large number of compounds.

15.2 Combinatorial Chemistry

It is a valuable means of drug discovery. It is a set of methods that authorize the synthesis of large numbers of chemical compounds employing several starting materials. Various chemical molecules like peptides, non-peptides, oligomers and small- molecules and natural products like organic molecules can be synthesized through this combinatorial chemistry. Each combinatorial approach has its own unique high throughput screening. The foremost advantage of combinatorial chemistry is the quick synthesis of original molecules. The use of combinatorial library depend on the particular structures and the objectives for which the library is to be tested. If the particular structure that would serve the anticipated need is known in advance, then a flourishing compound library would only need to have one substance in it. However, if one has just a general idea of the type of structure that would be serviceable, the library will have promising compounds, but still, be finite in number. The quantitative bioassay or screening of pure substances will allow one to select the most nearly perfect embodiment.

15.3 Solid-Phase Synthesis

Solid-phase synthesis is one of the most potent methods for the development of large compound libraries. Several advancements in solid-phase synthesis methodologies have been made in recent years.

15.4 Complex Multistep Synthesis on Solid Supports

15.4.1 Natural and Unnatural Oligomers

A number of synthetic techniques that have been used for the synthesis of libraries of small organic molecules were initially acquired for the chemical synthesis of biopolymers. A substantial amount of research has been done on the required activating protocols and the vast array of protecting groups that are required for the synthesis of large (20-100 steps) biopolymers in soaring yields and purities. The major classes of biopolymers, peptides, oligosaccharides, oligonucleotides, and unnatural oligomers have been chemically synthesized on support.

15.4.2 Array Technology

DNA microarrays can be used to map the expression patterns of thousands of genes in parallel, generating clues to gene function that can aid to identify suitable targets for the therapeutic intervention. They can also be used to monitor changes in gene expression in response to drug treatments [Figure 15.1].

Methodology

An appropriate enzymatic activity, preferably the rate-limiting step in the pathway, is identified and purified, most often from animal tissues. The refined enzyme is then screened against collections of structurally diverse small molecules. Finally, medicinal chemists work at optimizing the lead compounds bestowing desirable properties such as bioavailability and eliminating undesirable features such as target enzymes. DNA microarrays can be practiced for both genotyping and estimating mRNA levels. The DNA microarrays rapidly generate information essential for the identification and validation of innovative therapeutic targets.

The most engaging application of microarrays is in the study of differential gene expression in disease. Other techniques depend on either DNA sequencing or PCR-based differential display methods-these routines are complicated and often insensitive, e.g., rheumatoid tissue was recently analyzed using a microarray of about 100 genes known to have a role in inflammation.

Microarrays are potentially powerful tools for investigating the mechanism of drug action. In the long term, microarrays will contribute to the analysis of metabolic pathways such as the induction of cytochrome

P450 detoxifying enzymes for which new signaling pathways are being identified. They will also be used to delineate and predict adverse events, such as undesirable upregulation of liver enzymes.

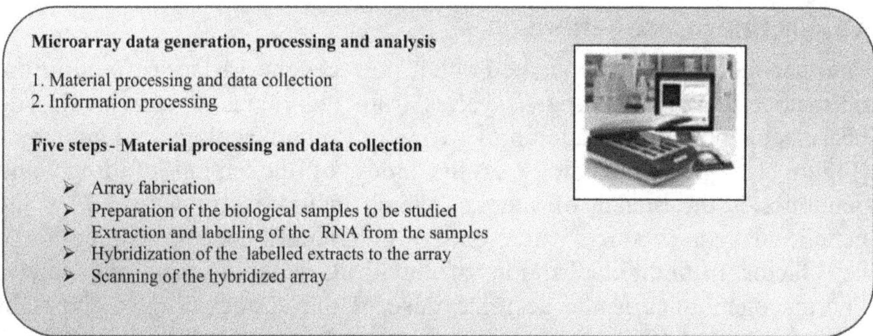

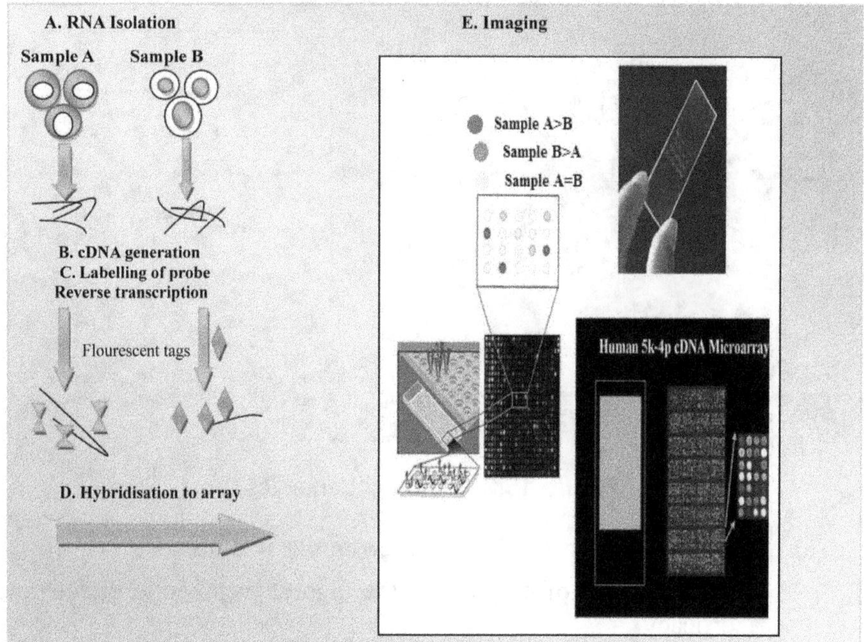

Figure 15.1 DNA microarrays technology.

15.4.3 Proteomics

Proteomics is an advantageous technique, and it may prove a better tool for drug discovery and development. The proteome is the complete set of proteins that are made and customized by an organism or system. Proteomics is an interdisciplinary field that has provided benefits to the genetic information of the Human Genome Project. Proteomics also gives advantage to various scientific researches. It provides information about protein structure, composition, and pattern. It is an essential component of functional genomics. Proteomics is mainly useful for the analysis of protein, purification of protein and mass spectrometry.

15.4.4 Pharmacogenomics

Pharmacogenomics is concerned about how genetic variations modify the ultimate effect of the drug. It varies from individual to individual. The pharmacogenomics is made up of two words: pharmacology and genomics [Figure 15.2]. Pharmacology is the study of the action of drugs and genomics is the branch of genetics which includes a review of how the genetic makeup produces variation. An individual's genetic makeup is the key factor in individualization of the drug with efficacy and safety. Pharmacogenomics is the accurate dose of the correct drug to the right patient at an exact time.

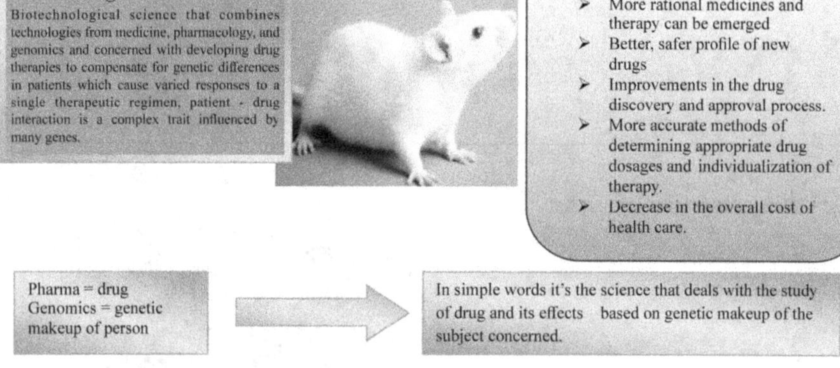

Figure 15.2 Pharmacogenomics.

(a)   Potential benefits of pharmacogenomics include

- Development of drugs with the highest therapeutic effects and efficacy.

- Drugs can be prescribed based on a patient's genetic profile.

- Prescription writing sometimes is based on trial and error method. Pharmacogenomics can combat the adverse drug reaction.

- Dosage calculation is mainly based on body weight and sex, but if it would be based on the genetic makeup of the individual, it can minimize the chance of overdosage.

- Vaccines made of genetic material could activate the immune system to have all the benefits of existing vaccines but with reduced risks of infections.

Pharmacogenomics is currently being used

- For the treatment of cardiac, respiratory, psychiatric situations and cancer.

- To know about the pharmacokinetics of the drug.

(b) Limitation of Pharmacogenomics include

- Multiple genes are likely to be involved in how someone reacts to a drug, making targeting drugs very complicated.

- Cataloging of the small variations in everyone's genes that may impact drug metabolism or how the condition develops is very challenging and time-consuming.

- The interactions with other drugs and environmental factors will need to be determined before any inferences are made about the genetic influence on how the drug is working.

15.5 Pharmacogenomics in Practice

15.5.1 Genetic Drug-Response Profiles

Rapid sequencing and genotyping of single nucleotide polymorphisms (SNPs) have a notable role in correlating sequence variations with heritable clinical phenotypes of drug or xenobiotic responses. Some drugs operate by adhering to the receptor on the surface of or within body cells. Variation in the genes that code for the receptors may mean that some people may present receptors that do not interact well with the drug. For example, some people have a lack of response to the drug salbutamol, used in the treatment of asthma, due to genetic variation in the gene that codes a receptor on the surface of smooth muscle cells lining airways of the lungs.

15.5.2 Drug Discovery and Development

The classification of all genes and, eventually, the study of all protein variants that cause, contribute to, or modify a disease, will direct to new 'druggable' and 'nondrugable' targets, prognostic markers of disease states or severity-of-disease knowledge. The discovery of genes and proteins that are linked in the pathogenesis of disease permits the identification of new drug targets and pledges to change the field of medicine in the future.

15.5.3 Drug Metabolism

The process of break down and the metabolism of drugs in the body can also be reshaped by their genetic information. For example, genetic polymorphism has been identified for many drug-metabolizing enzymes, like the cytochrome P450 (CYP450) enzymes. This may be responsible for different population phenotypes of individuals who have metabolism capacities ranging from extremely poor to fast. Genetic differences in drug metabolism are also an important consideration in the assessment of ocular toxicity caused by drugs and other environmental pollutants.

References

- Pavia, R. M., Sawyer, T. K., Moos, H. W. The generation of molecular diversity. Bioorganic Med Chem Lett.1993; 3:387-396.

- Lam, S. K., Li, X., Liu, R. Combinatorial chemistry in drug discovery. CurrOpin Cell Biol. 2017; 38:117-126.

- Belle, D. J., and Singh, H.Genetic factors in drug metabolism. Am Fam Physician. 2008; 77:1553-1560.

Chapter 16

Research Methodology

16.1 Research

Research means to search, to know and to find out a new conclusion. It is an organized and a reproducible process which identifies and defines problems, within specified boundaries. It employs a well-designed method to collect the data and analyses the results. Research can make progress in a particular field. Essential characteristics of the research are:

- Problem-solving should be systematic.
- Research is mostly consistent procedures that can be repeated or used by others.
- Empirical, most of the times decisions are based on data collected.
- Reductive, it can be performed in simplified form, and it examines a small sample that can be generalized to a larger population.
- Research should be replicable, so the results can be found by repeating the procedure.

16.1.1 Objectives of Research

- To obtain new facts.
- To confirm and test essential facts.
- To investigate an event or process.
- To make new scientific tools, concepts, and theories.
- To answer and understand scientific and non-scientific problems.
- To discover solutions to scientific, nonscientific and social problems.
- To solve the problems occurring in our everyday life.

16.2 Research Methods

Research methods are various techniques, systematic arrangements, algorithms, etc. practiced in research. All the manoeuvre used in research during a research study are referred to as research methods. It includes analytical procedures, experimental studies, numerical schemes, statistical approaches, etc. Research methods comprise a collection of data and to find a resolution to the problem. For the most part, scientific research techniques give interpretations dependent on gathered realities, estimations and perceptions and not on thinking alone. They acknowledge just those clarifications which can be checked by experiments.

16.2.1 Types of Research Methods

There are many different types of research methods. These are also known as research designs.

(a) **Experiment:** Subjects are arbitrarily allocated to various groups being contemplated. Groups are treated with distinctively in one or a couple of specific ways, the independent variable. Behavior resulting from this treatment difference is measured which is the dependent variable. If one of the groups treated with different treatments and other group does not, usually the treated group is called the experimental group, and other groups are called control groups or vehicle-treated group. Conditions other than the independent variable are held as constant as possible for all groups. These continuous conditions are called controls. If subjects are their control group, that is, they receive both research treatments; the design is called a within-subjects experiment. Inferences can be taken to show a cause and logical results relationship between the independent and dependent variables. Because of this, the experiments are in a class by itself, and it is an exceptional type of research procedure.

(b) **Correlational study:** A correlational study illustrates the relationship between two variables. Data are summarized as correlation coefficients. Strength and direction (positive or negative) of relationships can be shown by correlational studies, but indispensable links remain an open question.

(c) **Longitudinal study:** A longitudinal report pursues a gathering of information from a similar subject over and again for a range of time, the group made out of related individuals over the time of the life expectancy. Longitudinal examinations sometimes cover a concise time frame for a few weeks or sometimes for quite a prolonged time, for example, the entire life expectancy.

(d) **Cross-sectional study:** It is also called transverse studies. A cross-sectional examination usually examines groups of different people belonging to diverse age groups as a means of investigating behavioral development during a part or all of life. These investigations can generally be performed more effortlessly and rapidly than longitudinal examinations, yet the subsequent information might be of lower quality. All the more seldom, the term cross-sectional might be utilized to portray studies that divide and examine segments of society conditioned on factors other than age, for example, income, educational level or family estimate.

(e) **Case study:** A case investigation includes widespread observation of the few individuals. Information gathering may incorporate observing behavior, meetings and record searching. Case studies may be retrospective and/or perspective. As a rule, case investigations are employed where the activity or circumstance is rare than other methods, including larger groups of participants, which are not possible.

16.3 Research Methodology

Research methodology is a precise method to solve a problem. It is an exploration of concentrate on how research is to be done. For the most part, the strategies by which scientists approach their work of depicting, clarifying and their hypothesis are called research methodology. It is additionally portrayed as the investigation of methods by which information is picked up. Its point is to give the work plan of research.

16.3.1 Importance of Research Methodology in the Research Study

Designing a research methodology is essential for research design. The researcher should know that even if the methods considered in two problems are the same, the methodology could be different. The researcher needs to understand not only the research methods necessary for the research carried out but also the methodology. For example, a researcher does not just need to know how to calculate the mean, variance and distribution function for a data set, how to find a solution of a physical system described by the mathematical model, how to determine the roots of algebraic equations and how to apply a particular method, and one must also know

- Which is a suitable method for the chosen problem?
- What is the order of accuracy of the result of a method?
- What is the efficiency of the method?

Consideration of these aspects constitutes a research methodology. On the other hand, research methodology is concerned with the explanation of the following:

- Why is a particular research study undertaken?
- How did one formulate a research problem?
- What types of data were collected?

- What particular method has been used?
- Why was a particular technique of analysis of data used?

16.3.2 Types of Research

Research is broadly classified into two main classes:

- Fundamental or basic research
- Applied research

(a) Fundamental or basic research

Basic research is an exploration of fundamental standards and explanations behind a particular event or process or phenomenon. It is also called theoretical research. It is identified with a natural phenomenon or relating to basic science. It isn't uncertain for taking care of any handy issues of prompt intrigue. It offers an efficient and profound knowledge into an argument and encourages the extraction of logical and consistent clarification and conclusion on it. Applied research relies on essential research for its results. Researchers working on applied research have to make use of the findings of basic research and explore the utility of them. Fundamental research leads to a new theory or a unique property of matter or even the existence of a new thing, the knowledge of which has not been known or reported earlier. For example, fundamental research on

- Identification of new planets or stars in our galaxy comes under fundamental research.
- Structure, contents, and functioning of various parts of the human body help us identify the basis for certain diseases.

(b) Applied Research

In applied research, specific problems are solved in well-known and accepted theories and principles. Most experimental research, case studies, and interdisciplinary research are permanently applied research. Applied research is useful for basic research. Research, the result of which has immediate application is also called applied research. This research is of practical use for the current activity. For example, research on social problems has immediate use. Applied research involves real-life research, such as research into increasing the efficiency of a machine, increasing the gain factor of producing material, controlling contamination, preparing vaccination against diseases, etc. They have immediate potential applications. Therefore, the central objective of applied research is to find a solution to a practical problem that justifies a solution for its immediate use, while fundamental research is aimed at finding information that has a broad base of applications and, therefore, adds new information to existing scientific knowledge. Difference between basic and applied research exist which is depicted in Table 16.1.

Table 16.1 Difference between basic and applied research

S. No.	Basic research	Applied research
1.	Seeks generalization	Studies individual or specific cases without the objective to generalize
2.	Aims at basic processes	Aims at any variable which makes the desired difference
3.	Attempts to explain why things happen	Tries to say how things can be changed
4.	Tries to get all the facts	Tries to correct the facts which are problematic
5.	Reports in technical language of the topic	Reports in common language

16.4 Selection of a Research Topic and Problem

The very first duty of research is a selection of research topics and issues. To choose an appropriate research topic is one of the most challenging part of research. Before selecting a research topic and a problem, the researchers should keep the following points in mind.

- The topic should be novel.
- Researchers interest in the topic is necessary.
- The facility to perform research must be there.
- The topic should not be chosen by compulsion.

16.4.1 Identification of a Research Topic and Problems

Some sources of identification of a research topic and issues are:

- Theory of one's interest
- Daily problems
- Technological changes
- Recent trends
- Unexplored areas
- Discussion with experts and research supervisor

Choosing a topic of current interest or recent trends provides bright and promising opportunities for young researchers to get a post-doctoral fellowship, position in leading institutions in our nation and abroad. In each subject, several topics are not explored in detail even though the problem was considered by scientists a long time ago. For instance, string hypothesis, quantum registering, nanoparticles, quantum cloning, and quantum cryptography and gene immunology are interesting points and are in preliminary stages.

The supervisors and experts are working on one or a few fields over a long time, and they are the specialists in the area considered and well versed with the development and current status of the field. Therefore, a young researcher can make utilization of their skill in knowing different conceivable issues in the subject, the solving of which give opportunities in all aspects.

16.4.2 Definition and Formulation of a Problem

After identifying a problem, to solve it, it has to be defined and appropriately formulated. For this purpose, one can execute the following.

- State the problem in questionnaire form or an equivalent form
- Specify the problem in detail and precise terms
- List the assumptions made
- Remove the ambiguities, if any, in the statement of the problem
- Examine the feasibility of a particular solution

Characterizing the problem is more critical than its solution. It is a significant piece of the research study and not to be portrayed in a hurry. Finally, the researcher must ensure that the vital experimental setup and materials to perform genuine research work are accessible in the office where research work is to be carried out. Without these, if the researcher-initiated the work and had experienced certain phases of work or went through a couple of years in the issue then to finish the task, he/she would be compelled to purchase the materials and instruments from his/her reserve funds.

16.5 Literature Survey

After defining a problem, the researcher has to do a literature survey connected with the problem. The literature survey is a collection of research publications, books and other documents related to the defined problem. It is important to know whether the described problem has already been solved, the status of the issue, strategies that are valuable to research the problem and other related details. One can survey:

- The reputed journal which publishes research or review paper in the same area of research.

- Review articles related to the topic chosen.
- Advanced level books on the chosen topic.
- Proceedings of conferences, workshops, etc.
- Internet.

No research shall be complete unless we make use of the knowledge available in books, journals, and the internet. A review of the literature in the area of research is a preliminary step before attempting to plan the study.

16.5.1 Importance of a Literature Survey

Literature survey helps us

- Sharpen the problem, reformulate it or even leads to defining other closely related issues.
- Get a proper understanding of the problem chosen,
- To acquire appropriate theoretical and practical knowledge to investigate the issue,
- Show how the problem under study refers to the previous research studies,
- Know whether the proposed problem had already been solved,
- To speculate the possible mechanism of action for proposed study and
- To co-relate novel aspects or possible involvement of our body systems with the proposed study which were not explored before.

A literature survey provides relevant information about the problem. Various ideas can be taken from the literature survey. Apart from the literature directly connected with the problem, the literature that is connected with similar problems is also useful. It figures the issue in an obvious manner. A survey of past work encourages us to know the result of those examinations where similar issues were solved. It can help us design methodology for the present work. We can also investigate the essential connections with the different patterns and stages in the chosen topic and familiarize them with trademark statutes, ideas, and interpretations. Further, it can help us formulate a satisfactory structure for the research proposal.

16.6 Research Hypothesis

Researchers do not carry out work without any aim or expectation. Research is not about doing something and presenting what is done. Every research problem is undertaken aiming at specific outcomes. That is, before starting actual work such as performing a theoretical experiment calculation or numerical analysis, we expect specific findings from the study. The expectations form the hypothesis is scientifically reasonable predictions. They are often stated in terms of if-then sentences in specific coherent structures. Speculation should provide what we hope to discover in the chosen research problem. In other words, the expected or proposed solutions based on available data and tentative explanations constitute the hypothesis.

Hypothesizing is done only after a survey of relevant literature and learning the present status of the field of research. It can be formulated based on previous research and observation. To develop a hypothesis, the researcher should attain enough knowledge on the topic of research and problem. In formulating a hypothesis construct operational definitions of variables in the research problem.The hypothesis is due to an intelligent guess or for motivation which is to be tried in the examination work thoroughly through a suitable strategy. The testing of the hypothesis leads to an explanation of the associated phenomenon or event.

16.6.1 Criteria of a Good Hypothesis

An acceptable hypothesis should fit in the theoretical clarity. Further, it should be testable. It should be stated suitably so that it can be tested by the investigation. When data are analyzed, initially made hypothesis may be incorrect. In this case, it has to be revised. It is important to state the research problem hypothesis in a research report. If a hypothesis which stands the experiments and provides the required facts to make it acceptable then after continual verification the hypothesis may become a theory.

16.6.2 Tests of Hypothesis

Hypothesis test determines the validity of the presumption to pick between two different hypotheses about the estimation of a populace parameter. Hypothesis testing helps to decide based on sample data, whether a hypothesis about the population is probably going to be valid or false. Statisticians have developed several tests of the hypothesis or tests of significance like:

- Parametric tests or standard tests of hypothesis
- Non-parametric tests or distribution-free test of the hypothesis

Parametric tests are those statistical tests in which assumptions of the parameters are taken from the same parent population such as mean-variance etc. Presumptions like perceptions originate from a normal population; the sample size is large, assumptions about the population parameters like mean, fluctuation, etc. must hold great before parametric tests can be utilized. But there are situations when the researcher cannot or does not want to make such assumptions, in such situations, we use statistical methods for testing hypotheses which are called non-parametric tests because such tests do not depend on any assumption about the parameters of the parent population. Besides, most non-parametric tests assume only nominal or ordinal data, whereas parametric tests require measurement equivalent to at least an interval scale.

(a) Parametric tests

The different parametric tests are discussed below. All these tests are based on the assumption of normality, i.e., the source of data is considered to be normally distributed.

(i) *z-test:* z-test is based on the normal probability distribution and is used for evaluating the significance of several statistical measures, particularly the mean. The important test measurement, z, is worked out and contrasted with its probable value at a predefined level of significance for deciding the significance of the measure concerned. This is the most frequently used test in research studies. This test is used even when binomial distribution or t-distribution is applicable on the presumption that such a distribution tends to approximate a normal distribution as 'n' becomes larger. z-test is generally used for comparing the mean of a sample to some hypothesized mean for the population in case of a large sample, or when the population variance is known. Besides, this test may be used for evaluating the significance of median, mode, the coefficient of correlation and several other measures.

(ii) *t-test*: *t-test* is based on t-distribution and is considered as an important test for evaluating the significance of a sample mean or for judging the significance of the difference between the means of two samples in case of the small sample when the population variance is not known. In the case of two samples that are related, we use a *paired t-test* (also known as difference test) for judging the significance of the mean of the difference between the two related samples. It can also be used for judging the significance of the coefficients of simple and partial correlations. The relevant test statistic, t, is calculated from the sample data and then compared with its probable value based on t-distribution at a specified level of significance for concerning degrees of freedom for accepting or rejecting the null hypothesis. It may be noted that the t-test applies only in the case of a small sample when the population variance is unknown.

(iii) *χ2* **(chi-square)** *test:* is based on chi-square distribution and a parametric test is used for chi-square test comparing a sample variance to a theoretical population variance.

(iv) *F-test:* is based on *F*-distribution and is used to compare the variance of the two independent samples. This test is also used in the context of analysis of variance (ANOVA) for judging the significance of more than two sample means at the same time. It is also used for judging the significance of multiple correlation coefficients.The test statistic, *F*, is calculated and compared with its probable value (to be seen in the *F*-ratio tables for different degrees of freedom for greater and smaller variances at a specified level of significance) for accepting or rejecting the null hypothesis.

(b) Nonparametric test

Tests of hypotheses with 'order statistics' or 'nonparametric statistics' or 'distribution-free statistics' are known as nonparametric or distribution-free tests. Following types of nonparametric test are discussed below:

(i) **Sign test:** The sign test is one of the easiest parametric tests. Its name comes from the fact that it is based on the direction of the plus or minus signs of observations in a sample and not on their numerical magnitudes.

(ii) **Fisher-Irwin test:** Fisher-Irwin test is a nonparametric test used in testing a hypothesis concerning no difference among two sets of data. It is employed to determine whether one can reasonably assume, for example, that two supposedly different treatments are different in terms of the results they produce.

(iii) **McNemer test:** McNemer test is one of the important nonparametric tests often used when the data happen to be nominal and relates to two related samples. As such this test is especially useful with before-after measurement of the same subjects. The experiment is designed for the use of this test in such a way that the subjects initially are divided into equal groups as to their favorable and unfavorable views about, say, any system. After some treatment, the same numbers of subjects are asked to express their views about the given system whether they favor it or do not favor it.

(iv) ***Wilcoxon Matched-pairs Test (or Signed Rank Test):*** In various research situations in the context of two-related samples (i.e., case of matched pairs such as a study of two similar machines or where some subjects are studied in the context of before-after experiment) when we can determine both direction and magnitude of the difference between matched values, we can use an important non-parametric test viz., Wilcoxon matched-pairs test. While applying this test, we first find the differences (*di*) between each pair of values and assign a rank to the differences from the smallest to the largest without regard to sign. The actual signs of each difference are then put to corresponding ranks, and the test statistic T is calculated which happens to be the smaller of the two sums viz., the sum of the negative ranks and the sum of the positive ranks.While using this test, we may come across two types of tie situations. One situation arises when the two values of some matched pair(s) are equal, i.e., the difference between values is zero in which case we drop out the pair(s) from our calculations. The other situation arises when two or more pairs have the same difference value in such cases we assign ranks to such pairs by averaging their rank positions.

(v) ***Rank sum tests:*** Rank sum tests are a whole family of the test, and mainly divided into two parts:

- ***Wilcoxon-Mann-Whitney test (or U-test):*** This is a very popular test amongst the rank-sum tests. This test is used to determine whether two independent samples have been drawn from the same population. It uses more information than the sign test or the Fisher-Irwin test. This test applied under very general conditions and requires only that the populations sampled are continuous.

- ***The Kruskal-Wallis test (or H test):*** This test is conducted in a way similar to the U test described above. This test is used to test the null hypothesis that 'k' independent random samples come from identical universes against the alternative hypothesis that the means of these universe are not equal. This test is analogous to the one-way analysis of variance, but unlike the latter, it does not require the assumption that the samples come from approximately normal populations or the universes having the same standard deviation.

16.7 Research Design

For scientific research one has to prepare a research design. It should indicate the various approaches to be used in solving the research problem, sources, and information related to the challenge and, time frame and the cost budget. Essentially, the research design creates the foundation of the entire research work. The design will help perform the chosen task effectively and in a systematic way. Once the research design is completed, the actual action can be initiated. The first step in the actual work is to learn the facts about the problem. Particularly, theoretical methods, numerical techniques, experimental techniques and other relevant data and tools necessary for the present study have to be collected and learned.

Not every theory, technique, and information on the topic of research need to be useful for a particular problem. A researcher has to identify and select materials that are useful to the present work. Further, the validity and utility of the information gathered should be tested before using them. Scientific research is based on precise mathematical, numerical and experimental methods. These sources have to be properly studied and judged before applying them to the problem of interest.

16.7.1 Important Concepts Relating to Research Design

Following are the various concepts related to the research design

(a) **Dependent and independent variables:** A concept that can take different quantitative values is called a variable. As such, concepts such as weight, height, income are all examples of variables. Qualitative phenomena (or attributes) are also quantified based on the presence or absence of the characteristics in question. The aspects that can assume quantitatively different values even in decimal points are called "continuous variables." But all the variables are not continuous. If they can only be expressed in integral values, they are non-continuous variables or in the statistical language 'discrete variables.' Age is an example of a continuous variable, but the number of children is an example of a non-continuous variable. If a variable depends on or is a consequence of the other variable, it is called a dependent variable and the variable that precedes the dependent variable is called an independent variable. For example, if we say that height depends on age, height is a dependent variable and age is an independent variable. Moreover, if in addition to depending on age, height also depends on the gender of the individual, so height is a dependent variable and age and gender are independent variables. Likewise, prefabricated films and lectures are examples of independent variables, while behavioral changes, which occur as a result of environmental manipulations, are examples of dependent variables. Suppose the researcher wants to verify the hypothesis that there is a relationship between the gains of children in social studies success and their concepts. In this case, the idea of self is an independent and social variable, the achievements of studies are a dependent variable. Intelligence can also influence social studies success, but because it is not related to the purpose of the study conducted by the researcher, it is called as an unknown variable. Any effect that is noticed in the dependent variable like the result of the unknown variable is technically described as an "experimental error". A study must always be designed in such a way that the effect on the dependent variable is completely attributed to the independent variable and not to any variable or unknown variables.

(b) **Extraneous variable:** Independent variables that are not related to the purpose of the study, but can affect the dependent variable are called unknown variables.

(c) **Control:** An important feature of a good research project is to minimize the influence of either effect of the different variable (s). The technical term "control" is used when we design the study to minimize the effects of external independent variables. In experimental investigations, the term 'Control' is used to refer to limit experimental conditions.

(d) **Confounding variables relationship:** Confounding means confusing. When the dependent variable is not free from the influence of unknown variable (s), it is said that the relationship between the dependent and independent variables is be confounded by an unknown variable (s).

(e) **Research hypothesis:** When a theoretical prediction or relationship must be proved by scientist's methods, it is called a research hypothesis. The research hypothesis is a predictive declaration that refers to an independent variable to a dependent variable. In general, a research hypothesis must contain, at least, an independent variable and a dependent variable. Predictive statements that should not be verified objectively or the relationships that are assumed but not tested are not called the research hypothesis.

(f) **Experimental and control groups:** In an experimental test when the group is exposed to the usual conditions, it is called 'control group,' but when the group is exposed to some new or special conditions are called "experimental groups." Under usual condition, group A can serve as a control group, and group B an experimental group. If both groups A and B are exposed to special study programs, both groups would be called "experimental" groups. "We can design studies that include only experimental groups or include both experimental and control groups.

(g) Treatments: The different conditions in which the experimental and control groups are located are generally known as "treatments." If we want to determine through experiment the impact of three different doses of antihypertensive drugs, in that case, the test three doses of the drug will be treated as three treatments.

(h) Experiment: The process of examining the truth of a research problem, it is known as an experiment. For example, we can experiment to examine the usefulness of a specific new drug. The experiments can be of two types: independent experiment and comparative experiment. If we want to determine the impact of new analgesics in relieving pain, it is a case of an independent experiment; but if we want to determine the impact of new analgesics and compare to the impact of standard analgesics, our experiment will be called as a comparative experiment. Often, we conduct comparative experiments when we talk about the design of experiments.

(i) Experimental unit(s): The predetermined plots or blocks, where different treatments are used, they are known as experimental units. These experimental units must be selected a lot carefully.

16.8 The Basic Principle of Experimental Design

Following are the basic principal of experimental design

- Replication
- Randomization
- Local Control

16.8.1 Principle of Replication

In this principle, all treatments are applied in many experimental groups. Therefore, the statistical accuracy of the experimental groups is increased. For example, suppose we are to examine the effect of two different anti-inflammatory drugs (NSAIDS) on albino rats, for this purpose, we may divide the animals into two groups having the same number of animals, and study the effect of individual drugs on each group of rats. We can then compare the effect of both drugs and conclude which one is better. But if we are to apply the principle of replication to these experiments, then we have to use several groups of rats (suppose ten groups, five groups for each drug). We can then collect the data of these two drugs and conclude by comparing the same. The result so obtained will be more accurate in comparison to the results obtained without applying the principle of replication. The principle of replication shows computational difficulty. For example, if an experiment requiring a two-way analysis of variance is designed according to the principle of replication, then it will require a three-way analysis of variance since replication itself may be a source of variation in the data.

16.8.2 Principle of Randomization

This principal indicates that we should design or plan the research in such a way that the variations caused by external factors can all be combined under the general heading of chance.

16.8.3 The Principle of Local Control

The Principle of local controlis another important principle of experimental designs. Under it, the external factor, the known source of variability, is made to vary deliberately over as wide a range as necessary and this needs to be done in such a way that the variability it causes can be measured and hence eliminated from the experimental error. This suggests that we should plan the experiment in a manner that we can perform a two-way analysis of variance, in which the total variability of the data is divided into three components attributed to, treatments (varieties of rice), the external factor (soil fertility) and experimental error.

This suggests we should plan the examination such that we can play out a two-way examination of change, in which the hard and fast changeability of the data is isolated into three sections credited to treatment (groupings of rice), the outside factor (soil lavishness) and preliminary goof.

16.9   Important Experimental Designs

Experimental design refers to the framework or structure of an experiment, and as such there are several experimental designs. We can classify experimental designs into the following groups:

16.9.1 Informal Experimental Designs

(a) **Before and after without control design:** In this model, a single test group is selected, and the dependent variable is measured before the treatment is introduced. Then the treatment is presented, and the dependent variable is again measured after the introduction of the treatment. The effect of treatment would be equal to the level of the phenomenon after treatment minus the level of the phenomenon before treatment [Figure 16.1].

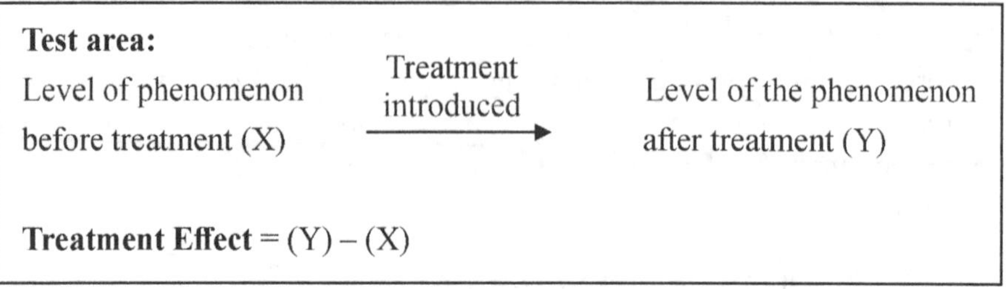

Figure 16.1 Before and after without control design.

(b) **After-only with control design:** In this design, two groups or areas (test area and control area) are selected, and the treatment is introduced just in the test area. The dependent variable is then measured in both areas simultaneously. The impact of the treatment is evaluated by subtracting the value of the dependent variable in the control area from its value in the test area [Figure 16.2]. The underlying assumption in this design is that the two areas are identical concerning their behavior towards the phenomenon considered. If this hypothesis is not correct, the possibility exists that the external variation enters the treatment effect. However, data can be collected in that design without the introduction of problems over time. In this sense, the design is superior to design before and after without control.

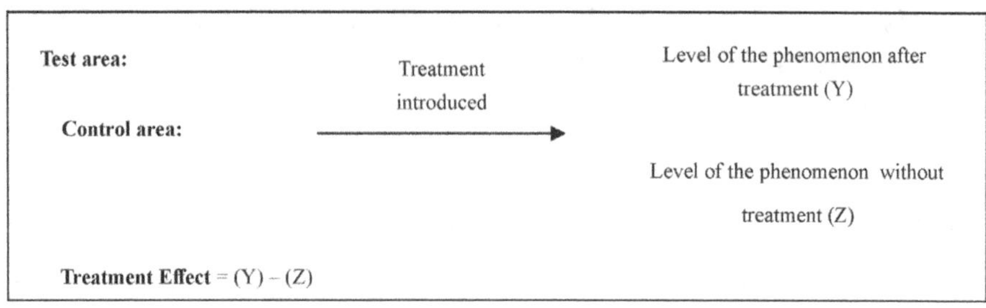

Figure 16.2 After-only with control design.

(c) **Before and after with control design**

In this design, two areas are selected, and the dependent variable is measured in both areas for an identical period before treatment. Then, the treatment is introduced into the test area, and the dependent variable is measured in both for an identical period. After the introduction of the treatment, the treatment effect is determined by subtracting the change in the dependent variable in the control area from that of the difference in the dependent variable in the test area [Figure 16.3].

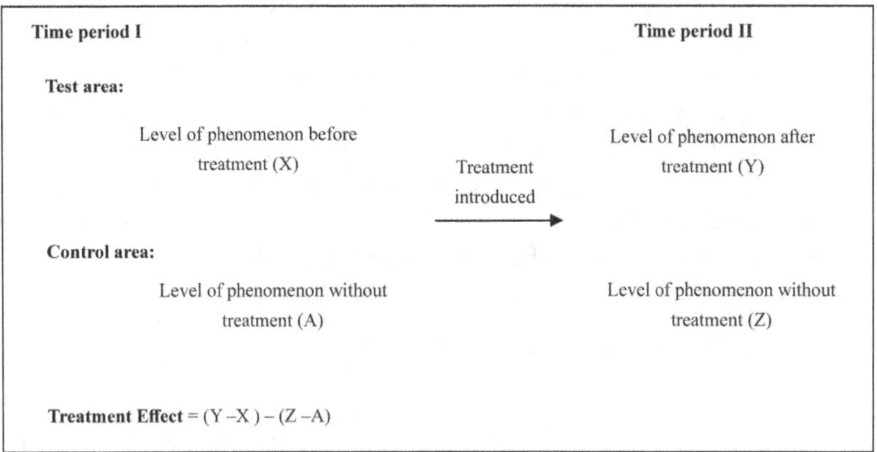

Figure 16.3 Before and after with control design.

This design is superior to the two previous designs for the simple reason that it avoids strange variations deriving both from the passage of time and from the non-comparability of the test and control areas. But sometimes, because of the lack of historical data, time or a comparable control area, we prefer to select one of the first two informal projects mentioned above.

16.9.2 Formal Experimental Designs

(a) **Completely randomized design (C.R. design):** It implies only two principles, namely the replication principle and the randomization principle of experimental models. It is the most straight forward possible design, and its analysis procedure is even simple. The essential feature of the design is that the subjects are randomly assigned to experimental treatments (or vice versa). For example, if we have 10 subjects and if we want to analyze 5 under treatment A and 5 under treatment B, the randomization process allows each possible group of 5 subjects selected from a set of 10 to have the same opportunity to be assigned to treatment A and treatment B. One-way analysis of variance (or unidirectional ANOVA) is used to analyze this project. Even irregular repetitions can work on this project. It provides the maximum number of degrees of error. This design is generally used when the experimental areas are homogeneous. Technically, when all the variations due to independent external factors are included under the heading of random variation, we refer to the design of the experiment as C.R.

(i)   Two groups simple randomized design: In a simple random project of two groups, first of all, the entire population is defined and a random sample is selected after the population. Furthermore, this design requires that the articles, after being randomly selected by the population, will be randomly assigned to the experimental and control groups (such as the assignment of articles to two groups is technically described as the principle of randomization). Therefore, this design produces two groups as representatives of the population [Figure 16.4].

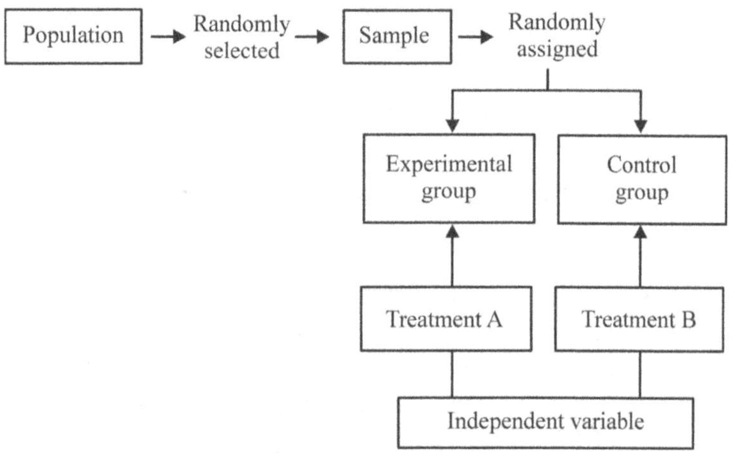

Figure 16.4 Two-group simple randomized design.

Because in the randomized design of the sample, the elements making up the example are randomly drawn from the same population and randomly assigned to the experimental and control groups, it is possible to conclude based on examples applicable for the specific population. The two groups (experimental and control groups) of this design are provided different treatments of the independent variable. This experimental design is quite common in research studies on behavioral sciences. The merit of such a project is that it is simple but the limitation of this is that the individual differences between those who perform the treatments are not eliminated, i.e., they do not control the external variable and, as such, the result of the experiment may not represent a correct image. Suppose the researcher wants to compare two groups of students who were randomly selected and randomly assigned. There are two different treatments, namely regular training and specialist training for the two groups. The researcher raises the hypothesis of higher profits for the group receiving specialized training. To determine this, test each group before and after practice, then compare the amount of gain for the two groups to accept or reject their hypothesis. This is an illustration of the randomized design of two groups, in which individual differences between students are randomized. But this does not control the differential effects of external independent variables.

(ii) **Random replications design:** The limitation of the two-group randomized design is usually eliminated within the random replications design. Each repetition is technically called a 'replication'. Random replication design serves two purposes viz., it provides controls for the differential effects of the extraneous independent variables and secondly, it randomizes any individual differences among those conducting the treatments. From the diagram Figure 16.5, it is clear that there are two populations in the replication project. The sample is randomized, for example, four experimental groups and four control groups. In general, the same number of elements is inserted into each group and the group cannot influence the outcome of the study. Variables related to both populations are randomly distributed between the two groups. Therefore, this random replication is a simple random project.

(b) **Randomized block design (R.B. design)** is an improvement over C.R. In the R.B. the principle of local control can be applied together with the other two principles of experimental projects. In the design of R.B., the subjects are first divided into groups, known as blocks, so that within each group the subjects are relatively homogeneous concerning some selected variables. The variable selected to group the subjects is the one that is considered to be related to the measures that must be obtained concerning the dependent variable. The number of subjects in a given block would be equal to the number of treatments and one subject in each block would be assigned randomly to each treatment.

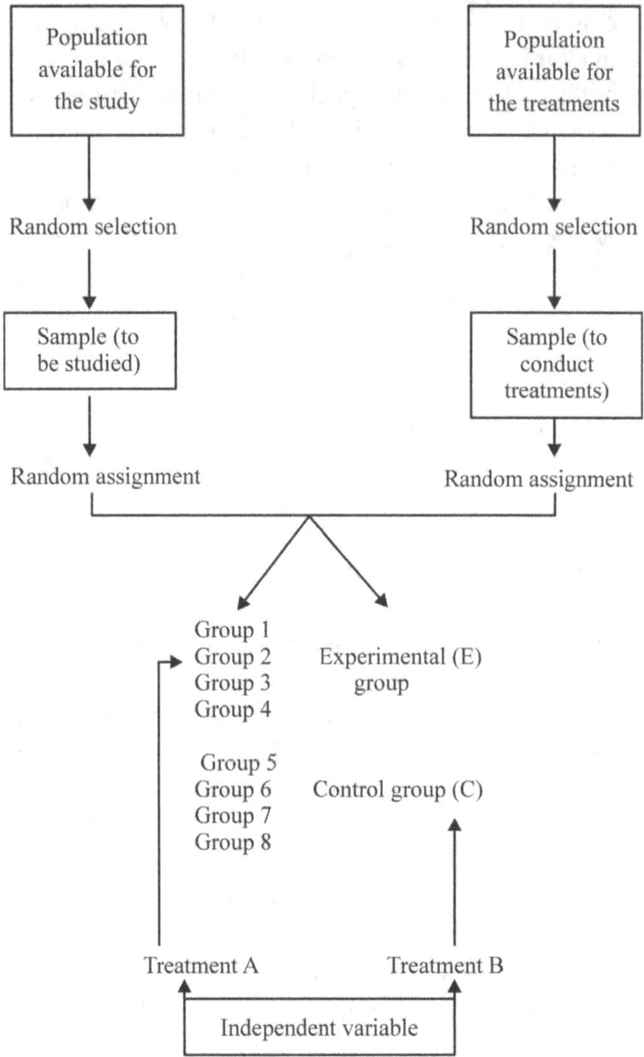

Figure 16.5 Random replication design.

(c) **Latin square design (L.S. design)** It is an experimental design widely used in agricultural research. The conditions under which agricultural research is conducted are different from those of other studies because nature plays an important role in agriculture. For example, an experiment must be done through which the effects of five different varieties of fertilizers are judged on the performance of a given crop, such as wheat. In this case, the variable fertility of the soil in different blocks in which the experiment being performed must be taken into consideration; otherwise, the results obtained may not be very reliable.

Outcome of study is not only due to the effect of fertilizers but also due to the effect of soil fertility. Likewise, there may be an impact of seed variation on yield. To overcome these difficulties, L.S. Design is used when there are two important external factors, such as variable soil fertility and seed variation.

(d) Factorial designs: Factorial designs are used in experiments where the effects of varying more than one factor are to be determined. They are especially important in several economic and social phenomena where usually a large number of factors affect a particular problem. This is classified into the

(i) Simple factorial designs: In the case of simple factorial drawings, we consider the effects of the variation of two factors in the dependent variable, but when an experiment is performed with more than two factors, we use complex factorial designs. The simple factorial design is also called the "factor design of two factors", while the complex factorial design is known as "multifactorial factorial design." The simple factorial design can be 2×2, or it can be the 3×4 or 5×3 or a similar type of simple factorial design.

(ii) Complex factorial designs: Experiments with more than two factors imply the use of complex factorial design simultaneously. A design that considers three or more independent variables are called complex factorial design. In the case of three factors with an experimental variable that has two treatments and two control variables, each of them that has two levels, the design used will be called complex factorial design.

16.10 Data Analysis

The data analysis is essential for a scientific study and for ensuring that we have all relevant data for making contemplated comparisons and analysis. The term analysis refers to the computation of certain measures along with searching for patterns of relationships that exist among data-groups. Thus, in the process of analysis, relationships or differences supporting or conflicting with original or new hypotheses should be subjected to statistical tests of significance to determine with what validity data can be said to indicate any conclusions.

16.10.1 Types of Analysis

Analysis, particularly in case of survey or experimental data, involves estimating the values of unknown parameters of the population and testing of hypotheses for drawing inferences. The analysis may, therefore, be categorized as

- Descriptive analysis
- Inferential analysis (also known as statistical analysis).

(a) **Descriptive analysis:** The descriptive analysis is basically the study of the distributions of a variable. This study provides profiles of companies, workgroups, people and other problems in any one of a multiple of features such as size, composition, efficiency, preferences, etc. This type of analysis can be compared to a variable or two variables or more than two variables. Following five types of analysis must be studied under descriptive analysis.

   (i) **Correlation analysis** tells about the common variation of two or more variables for determining the amount of correlation between two or more variables.

   (ii) **The causal analysis** deals with the study of how one or more variables influence changes in another variable. It is, therefore, a study of the functional relations existing between two or more variables. This analysis can be called a regression analysis. The causal analysis is considered relatively more important in the experimental investigations, while in most social and commercial investigations our interest is to understand and control the relationships between the variables with the determining causes per se and as such we consider the analysis of correlation, it is relatively more important.

   (iii) **The multivariate analysis** which may be defined as "all statistical methods which simultaneously analyze more than two variables on a sample of observations."

   (iv) **Multiple regression analysis** This analysis is adopted when the researcher has a dependent variable that should be a function of two or more independent variables. The objective of this analysis is to make a prediction on the dependent variable based on its covariance with all the independent variables involved.

   - Multiple discriminant analysis
   - This analysis is appropriate when the researcher has a single dependent variable that cannot be measured but can be classified into two or more groups based on some attributes. The objective

of this analysis is to predict the possibility of an entity belonging to a particular group based on different prediction variables.

- Multivariate analysis of variance *or multi-ANOVA*: This analysis is an extension of two way ANOVA, wherein the ratio of among group variance to within-group variance is worked out on a set of variables.

(v) **Canonical analysis:** this analysis can be used in the case of measurable and non-measurable variables to simultaneously provide a set of variables dependent on their covariance together with a set of independent variables.

(b) Inferential analysis

These are the various tests of importance to test hypotheses to determine what validity it can be said that the data indicate some conclusion. It is also concerned about the estimation of population values. It is mainly based on the inferential analysis that the interpretation task is performed (i.e., the task of drawing inferences and conclusions).

16.11 Statistics in Research

The role of statistics in research is to function as a tool in designing research, analyzing its data and drawing conclusions. Most research studies result in a large volume of raw data which must be suitably reduced so that the same can be read quickly and can be used for further analysis. The science of statistics cannot be ignored by any research worker, even though he/she may not have the occasion to use statistical methods in all their details and ramifications. Classification and tabulation, as stated earlier, achieve this objective to some extent, but we have to go a step further and develop specific indices or measures to summarise the collected/classified data. Only after this, we can adopt the process of generalization from small groups (i.e., samples) to the population.

16.11.1 Analysis of Variance (ANOVA)

Analysis of variance (ANOVA) is an advantageous technique in the fields of economics, biology, education, psychology, sociology, and business/ industry and research of several other disciplines. Multiple sample cases are analyzed by ANOVA. ANOVA measures differences amongst more than two sample means at the very same time. ANOVA can answer whether the samples were taken from a population with the same mean.

The ANOVA technique is essential in the context of all those situations where we want to compare more than two populations such as in comparing the yield of the crop from several varieties of seeds, the gasoline mileage of four automobiles, the smoking habits of five groups of university students and so on.

$$F = \frac{\text{Estimate of population variance based on between samples variance}}{\text{Estimate of population variance based on within samples variance}}$$

This value of F is to be compared to the F-limit for given degrees of freedom. If the F value we work out is equal or exceeds the F-limit value, we may say that there are significant differences between the sample means

(a) There are two types of ANOVA

- One way ANOVA
- Two way ANOVA

(i) One-way (or single factor) ANOVA:

In one-way ANOVA, only one factor is considered and then observes the reason for a said factor to be important is that several possible types of samples can occur within that factor.

Step 1: Obtain the mean of each sample, i.e., obtain

X1, X2, X3, ..., Xk

when there are k samples.

Step 2: Work out the mean of the sample means as follows:

$$\overline{\overline{X}} = \overline{X1} + \overline{X2} + \overline{X3} .... \overline{Xk} \, / \, \text{No. of samples (k)}$$

Step 3: Take the deviations of the sample means from the mean of the sample means and calculate the square of such differences which may be multiplied by the number of items in the corresponding example, and then obtain their total. This is known as the sum of squares for variance between the samples (or SS between). Symbolically, this can be written:

$$\text{SS between} = n1 \left(\overline{X1} - \overline{\overline{X}} \right) 2 + n2 \left(\overline{X2} - \overline{\overline{X}} \right) 2 + ... nk \left(\overline{Xk} - \overline{\overline{X}} \right) 2$$

Step 4: Divide the result of the (3) step by the degrees of freedom between the samples to obtain a variance or mean square (*MS*) between samples. Symbolically, this can be written:

MS between = SS between/ (k-1)

where $(k - 1)$ represents degrees of freedom (d.f.) between samples.

Step 5: Obtain the deviations of the values of the sample items for all the samples from similar means of the examples and calculate the squares of such differences and then obtain their total. This total is known as the sum of squares for variance within samples (or *SS* within). Symbolically this can be written:

$$\text{SS with in} = \Sigma\left(\overline{X}1i - \overline{\overline{X1}}\right)2 + \Sigma\left(\overline{X}2i - \overline{\overline{X2}}\right)2 + \Sigma\left(\overline{X}ki - \overline{\overline{Xk}}\right)2$$

i = 1, 2, 3,.....................

Step 6: Divide the result of step 5 by the degrees of freedom within samples to obtain the variance or mean square (*MS*) within samples.

MS within = SS within/ (n-k)

where $(n - k)$ represents degrees of freedom within samples,

n = total number of items in all the samples.

k = number of samples.

➢ For a check, the sum of squares of deviations for a total variance can also be worked out by adding the squares of deviations when the deviations for the individual items in all the samples have been taken from the mean of the sample means.

This total should be equal to the total of the result of the (3) and (5) steps explained above

i.e., *SS* for total variance = *SS* between + *SS* within.

The degrees of freedom for total variance will be equal to the number of items in all samples minus one $(n - 1)$. The degrees of freedom for between and within must add up to the degrees of freedom for a total variance, i.e.,

$$(n - 1) = (k - 1) + (n - k)$$

This fact explains the additive property of the ANOVA technique.

➢ Finally, *F*-ratio may be worked out as under:

F ratio = MS between /MS within

This report is used to judge whether the difference between different sample media is significant or is just a matter of sample fluctuations. For this purpose, we look at the table, providing the values of F for degrees of freedom given at different levels of significance. If they have calculated the value of F, as indicated above, is lower than the value of the table of F, the difference is considered negligible, i.e., due to chance and the null hypothesis that there is no difference between the exhibits means. In the case where the calculated value of F is equal to or higher than its table value, the difference is considered significant (meaning that the samples could not come from the same universe) and, therefore, the conclusion can be drawn. The higher the calculated value of F concerning the value of the table, the more precise and sure it can be on its conclusions.

(ii) Two way ANOVA

Two way ANOVA analyzes two factors simultaneously. For example, agricultural production can be classified based on different varieties of seeds and also based on different varieties of fertilizers used. A trading company can have its sales data classified based on different sellers and also based on sales in different regions. In a factory, the various units of a product produced during a certain period can be classified according to the different varieties of machines used and also according to the different degrees of labor. Such a two-way design can have repeated measurements of each factor or not have repeated values. The ANOVA technique is a bit different in the case of repeated measurements in which we also calculate the variation of the interaction.

ANOVA technique in the context of two-way design when repeated values are not there:

Since we do not have repeated values, we cannot directly calculate the sum of the squares inside the samples as we did in the case of one-way ANOVA. Therefore, we must calculate this residual variation or error by subtraction, once calculated the sum of the squares for the total variance and the variance between the varieties of treatment and the variation among the different types of the other treatment.

The various steps involved are as follows:

- ➢ Use the coding device, if the same simplifies the task.
- ➢ Take the total of the values of individual items (or their coded values as the case may be) in all the samples and call it T.
- ➢ Work out the correction factor as under:

$$\text{Correction factor} = (T)^2 / n$$

- ➢ Find out the square of all the item values (or their coded values as the case may be) one by one and then take its total. Subtract the correction factor from this total to obtain the sum of squares of deviations for a total variance. Symbolically, we can write it as the sum of squares of deviations for a total variance or total SS

$$X_{nj}^{2} = (T)^{2} / n$$

➤ Take the total of different columns and then get the square of each total column and divide these values into the square of each column by the number of elements in the respective column and take the total of the result thus obtained. Finally, subtract the correction factor from this total to get the sum of the squares of deviations for the variance between the columns or (SS between the columns).

➤ Take the total of several rows and then get the square of each row and divide these square values of each row by the number of elements in the corresponding row and take the total of the result thus obtained. Finally, subtract the correction factor from this total to get the sum of the squares of deviations for the variance between the rows (or SS between the rows).

➤ Sum of squares of deviations for residual or error variance can be worked out by subtracting the result of the sum of 5th and 6th steps from the result of the 4th step stated above. In other words,

Total $SS - (SS$ between columns $+ SS$ between rows$) = SS$ for residual or error variance.

➤ Degrees of freedom (d.f.) can be worked out as under:

d.f. for total variance $= (c \cdot r - 1)$

d.f. for variance between columns $= (c - 1)$

d.f. for variance between rows $= (r - 1)$

d.f. for residual variance $= (c - 1)(r - 1)$

where c = number of columns

r = number of rows

➤ ANOVA table can be set up in the usual fashion as shown in Table 16.2:

Table 16.2 Analysis of variance table for two-way ANOVA

Source of variation	Sum of squares (SS)	Degrees of freedom (d.f.)	Mean square (MS)	F-ratio
Between columns treatment	$\Sigma(T_j)^2/n_j-(T)^2/n$	$(c-1)$	SS between columns/(c–1)	MS between columns/ MS residual
Between rows treatment	$\Sigma(T_i)^2/n_i-(T)^2/n$	$(r-1)$	SS between rows/ (r–1)	MS between rows/ MS residual
Residual or error	Total SS – (SS between columns+ SS between rows)	$(c-1)(r-1)$	SS residual/ (c–1) (r–1)	
Total	$\Sigma X_{ij}^2 - (T)^2/n$	$(c.r-1)$		

In the table c = number of columns

r = number of rows

SS residual = Total SS – (SS between columns + SS between rows)

Therefore, the residual MS or the residual variance provides the basis for the F ratios related to the variation between the treatment of the column and the inter-row treatment. The residual MS is always due to the sampling fluctuations and therefore serves as a basis for the significance test. Both F ratios are compared with the respective table values, for certain degrees of freedom at a specific level of importance, as usual.

The relation F to the variation between the columns is equal to or greater than its table value, so the difference between the columns means that it is considered significant. In the same way, the relation F as for the variation between the lines can be interpreted.

References

- Kothari, C. R., 2004. Research Methodology: Methods and Techniques. Wiley Eastern, New Delhi. pp. 17-19.

- Shumway, R. H., Stoffer D. S. Time Series Analysis and Its Applications: With R Examples (Springer Texts in Statistics).4th Edition, Kindle Edition, Springer. 2017, pp-149-231.

- Patil, S., Mankar, A. Research Methodology: For Beginners. IJMS. 2(1), 2016, 1-6.

- Derntl, M. "Basics of research paper writing", IJTEL. 6 (2), 2014,105-123.